5 minute first aid for sport

British Red Cross

Caring for people in crisis

5 minute first aid for sport

Hodder Arnold

A MEMBER OF THE HODDER HEADLINE GROUP

Orders: Please contact Bookpoint Ltd, 130 Milton Park, Abingdon, Oxon OX14 4SB. Telephone: (44) 01235 827720, Fax: (44) 01235 400454. Lines are open from 9.00 to 18.00, Monday to Saturday, with a 24-hour message answering service. You can also order through our website www.hoddereducation.com

British Library Cataloguing in Publication Data
A catalogue record for this title is available from the British Library.

ISBN-10: 0 340 90464 X
ISBN-13: 9 780340 904640

First published	2005
Impression number	10 9 8 7 6 5 4 3 2 1
Year	2008 2007 2006 2005

Typeset by Transet Limited, Coventry, England.
Printed in Great Britain for Hodder Arnold, a division of Hodder Headline, 338 Euston Road, London NW1 3BH, by Cox & Wyman Ltd, Reading, Berkshire.

contents

acknowledgements

The authors would like to pay special thanks to Charlotte Hall, Catherine Jones, Genevieve Okech and Naomi Safir.

preface

The British Red Cross, as part of the International Red Cross and Red Crescent Movement, is the world's largest first-aid training organization. With over 180 Red Cross societies worldwide, we endeavour to make first-aid knowledge and skills accessible to individuals, families, schools and the wider community.

You never know when someone may need your help but it is highly likely that when called on to provide emergency first aid it will be to someone close to you such as a friend or a member of your own family. Therefore, we have produced the *Five-minute First Aid* series in order to give you the relevant skills and confidence needed to be able to save a life and help an injured person, whatever your situation.

We appreciate that it is difficult to find time in hectic lifestyles to learn first-aid skills. Consequently, this series is designed so that you can learn and absorb each specific, essential skill that is relevant to you in just five minutes, and you can pick up and put down the book as you wish. The features throughout the book will help you to reinforce what you have learnt and will build your confidence in applying first aid.

This book is divided into five-minute sections, so that you can discover each invaluable skill in just a short amount of time.

one-minute wonder

One-minute wonders ask and answer the questions that you might be thinking as you read.

key skills

The key-skills features emphasize and reiterate the main skills of the section – helping you to commit them to memory and recall them when called upon to do so.

summary

Summary sections summarize the key points of the chapter in order to further consolidate your knowledge and understanding.

self-testers

The self-testers ensure that you have learnt the most important facts of the chapter. They will give you an indication of how much you are absorbing as you go along and help to build your confidence. (Note: some of the multiple choice questions may have more than one possible answer!)

We hope that this book will give you the opportunity to learn the most important skills you will ever need in a friendly, straightforward way, and that it prepares you for any first-aid situation that you may encounter.

introduction

Sport is about fun, enjoyment, camaraderie and getting fit or maintaining your fitness levels. Some of us are very competitive when participating in sports and the will to win dominates the activity, while for others the taking part is what matters. Whatever your approach to sport, the one thing that is common to all activities is that it places additional demands on the body both mentally and physically. However, the last thing we want to think about when putting the golf clubs in the boot of the car or the jersey and boots in the kit bag is that we may get injured or become unwell. Inevitably accidents do happen – thankfully many of these injuries and illnesses are minor and are easily treated but others are more serious and require a more skilled response.

As first-aid professionals, we are becomingly increasingly aware of the importance of the care a person receives before he arrives in hospital – there are some important things that you can do on the pitch, on the court, on the piste or on the course before the ambulance arrives or you get professional medical advice. Some of these things may help the person recover more quickly, on other occasions your actions may make the person more comfortable while waiting for the ambulance, and there may be the time when what you do may just save the person's life.

We have written this book in a way that gives you practical advice on how to respond to a wide variety of sports-related injuries and conditions. We recognize that there is a lot to remember so we have included a summary of the advice at the end of each chapter. Additionally, we have answered the more common questions we have been asked about first aid over the years. At the end of each chapter you will find a section that will allow you to test yourself on what you have learnt.

While we are confident that this book contains the key advice about what to do in more common emergency situations, this is only of value if you are prepared to step forward and use your newly-acquired skills and knowledge – that's what being a team member is all about.

For convenience and clarity, we use the pronoun 'he' when referring to the first aider or injured person.

1

what to do in an emergency

Players and spectators do not often consider the possibility of an emergency occurring during a sporting activity. However, organizers of events must take this into consideration because, by its very nature, an emergency is unexpected and it is important to know what to do and to have plans for such an incident. Contingency plans should include how to stop play quickly as this can sometimes be difficult, for example at a horse racing or motorbike race meeting.

how to deal with an emergency

When you find yourself dealing with an unexpected emergency it is important to make sure that you do not put yourself in danger so if there is obvious danger such as galloping horses or traffic it is important to deal with this first. It is also important to keep bystanders away from the danger.

Sometimes it can be dangerous for you to help a person. Examples of danger that would prevent you from approaching the scene include smoke, fire, toxic fumes or hazardous chemicals. Toxic chemicals are commonly kept around a swimming pool so be aware of the possibility of contamination. Falling masonry and bomb blasts can also be a danger. Around water, swirling or deep water or flooding (especially if you are a non-swimmer) can be a potential hazard, and when skating, iced-over ponds are a hazard especially when the ice is starting to melt.

***one-minute** wonder*

Q Is it safe to go into an iced-over pond in order to save a stranded person?

A It is very unsafe to do this because if you fall into the water, hypothermia very quickly takes hold and you will be unable to help and you will have put yourself in danger too. It is much better to help from the side of the pond.

If there is no serious danger and you think it is safe to approach an incident, try to find out what has happened and how many people are involved.

specific incidents

vehicle crashes

Crashes are a potential hazard at motor sports such as motor cross, motor racing or rallying. If you come across a crash and it is safe to approach, alert the emergency services. Usually at such a crash you will need police, fire and ambulance services. Send bystanders to warn other drivers.

Stabilize any vehicles involved in the crash by switching off the ignition and applying the handbrake. Make sure you look for all the injured people as someone may have been thrown from a moving vehicle.

one-minute wonder

Q If I am treating a person in the middle of a race track, should I move him first?

A It is important that you do not move the person until you have assessed his injuries. If you suspect a back or neck injury you certainly must not move him – instead ask bystanders and marshals to stop the race and stop any vehicles from passing the scene.

fire

A fire can occur at any sporting venue so it is good practice to take time to familiarize yourself with your surroundings and make sure you know where the fire exits are.

If you are aware of a fire or of smoke, sound the fire alarm and warn as many people as possible in the area of the fire. Remember that fire and smoke can spread quickly.

If the fire alarm sounds it is essential to think quickly to evacuate the building. There are some general principles to follow – if the fire is small and you have a fire blanket or fire extinguisher you can try to put out the fire, but do not try for longer than 30 seconds and if the fire has taken hold do not try to put it out. Do not use any lifts and close all doors behind you. Do not open a door without first touching the door handle. If it is hot this indicates that there is a fire behind the door so do not open it – find another escape route. When leaving a building, walk quickly but do not run and if you have to cross a smoke-filled area stay close to the ground where there will be the least smoke. If a fire traps you go into a room with a window and shut the door. Open the window and shout for help. If you are able to reach the ground outside the building from the window, escape by going out feet first and lowering yourself onto the ground. Call the emergency services as soon as possible.

key skills

In the event of a fire:

- sound the alarm
- warn any people in the vicinity of the fire
- use a fire extinguisher to fight the fire
- after 30 seconds get out and close the doors behind you.

one-minute wonder

Q I thought that if you press the fire alarm it automatically calls the fire services but you advise I call them after I have pressed the fire alarm. Why is this necessary?

A The main purpose of a fire alarm is to warn the occupants of a fire and to evacuate the building. In some buildings there is a direct link to the fire service, however, in most cases a call will have to be made. If in doubt call the emergency services.

how to put out the flames if a person is on fire

If a person runs from a burning building with his clothes on fire you should:

- **STOP** the person from moving around as this will fan the flames
- **DROP** the person to the ground
- **WRAP** the person in a non-flammable material
- **ROLL** the person slowly along the ground to extinguish the flames.

water

Water is a potential hazard with any water sports. The main dangers relating to rescue from water are that the water may be cold and deep and there may be strong underwater currents, so when attempting to rescue someone from water it is very important that you do not put yourself at risk. It is best to rescue from the water's edge, making sure that you do not get pulled into the water. You can throw a rope or float to the person or reach out with a stick or branch if close to the edge of the water.

If you have to go into the water, wade rather than swim and do not go out of your depth. Make sure the person's head is out of the water and then drag him to the side. Do not lift the person unnecessarily but try to shield him from cold wind to prevent any further hypothermia.

electricity

The combination of water from showers and electricity sockets for hair dryers is a potential danger in changing rooms so you should be aware of the safety of the electrical supply. The majority of injuries caused by an electric current are due to faulty switches or appliances.

If someone is electrocuted don't touch him until all the electricity is off because if you contact the current you too will be electrocuted. If it is not possible to turn the electricity off, separate the person from the electrical source. To do this, stand on some dry insulating material such as a book or folded newspaper then, using something made of wood such as a broom, push the electrical source away from the person or the person away from the source. If this is still not possible, carefully loop some rope around the person's ankles and pull him away from the electrical source.

one-minute *wonder*

Q Can I use a metal pole to isolate the person from the electricity?

A No, because metal will conduct electricity and you will receive a shock. You must use a material that does not conduct electricity such as wood or paper.

key skills

Do not touch a person with a possible electrical injury until the current has been switched off or the source of the electricity has been moved from the person. Remember that water conducts electricity.

calling for help

Everyone, when faced with an emergency, feels some anxiety so it is a good idea to shout loudly to see if anyone can come to help. Usually at a sporting event there will be other people around. You will feel less anxious if you have help and you may also be faced with doing several tasks at once, such as securing and maintaining safety of the scene, calling for the emergency services, bringing first-aid equipment, maintaining a person's privacy or helping with first aid, especially if there are lots of injured people, so another pair of hands will always be useful. The increased availability of mobile telephones makes it easier to call for help.

Bystanders can be helpful if they are given clear instructions and if they are kept busy as this may reduce the panic and confusion that always surrounds a significant emergency. You should give helpers clear instructions and if you are the most experienced first aider present, take control. Tell others you are trained to give first aid and if other first aiders come forward ask them to help to locate and assess the injured people. Try to maintain a clear picture of what is happening so that you can pass on accurate information to the emergency services and if you ask a bystander to call the emergency services check that it has been done.

calling the emergency services

To call the emergency services in the UK you must dial 999. In the EU, the emergency number is 112.

In the UK everyone knows it is possible to contact the fire, police and ambulance services using 999 but people are often surprised to know that you can also contact the mountain rescue, fell rescue, cave rescue and coastguard using this number.

When you dial 999 or 112, you will be asked which service you need. If it is a serious emergency with several injured people or if safety is a problem, you may need fire, police and ambulance services.

The operator will ask you for some information about the emergency, so it is important to have some answers before you phone, such as your location and your phone number. You will also be asked to give an indication of the type and seriousness of the emergency, the number of people injured and whether or not there are any dangers such as chemicals or toxic fumes.

key skills

In most emergency situations, an early call to the emergency services is key. Try and gather as much information as you can about the injured person or persons and be clear about the location of the accident.

one-minute wonder

Q Is it true that the ambulance service gives priority to some calls and not to others?

A The ambulance service responds to all 999 calls as soon as possible. In some cases the ambulance service will dispatch the closest available paramedic. The paramedic will not always arrive in an ambulance – he may be in a car, on a motorbike or a bicycle. Sometimes a community first responder will be first on the scene.

managing an incident

It is important to adopt a systematic approach to any emergency in order to give people the best chance of survival. Make sure you are clear in your mind about how to use bystanders, how to access the emergency services and how to assess people for injuries.

assessing the scene

Make sure you know how many people are involved. If you have to deal with two or more injured people, always treat the quiet person first as he may be unconscious and will need your immediate attention. You can be sure that if a person is shouting or crying out in pain he is not unconscious. Ask helpers to remove any people with minor injuries from the scene to improve access to those with serious injuries. Perform a primary survey (see below) on anyone who is unconscious and treat him first using your life-saving skills if necessary. Then treat conscious people with serious injuries and then those with minor injuries.

the primary survey

The aim of the primary survey is to establish if a person is conscious and breathing so that you can decide if life saving is needed. Making sure it is safe to do so, start by finding out whether the person is conscious or unconscious. You do this by shouting loudly at the person – if you know the person's name use it. If you are assessing an adult you can shake the shoulders gently and if dealing with a child you should tap the shoulder.

If the person is unconscious and you have not already shouted for help do so now. Then you should open the airway, check for breathing, and if breathing is present, check for other life-threatening injuries such as severe bleeding and place the person in the recovery position (see Chapter 2, page 31).

the secondary survey

Having completed the primary survey and decided no life-saving action is required you can perform a secondary survey. The aim of the secondary survey is to find out more about the person's condition so that the correct first aid can be administered.

You should find out more about the incident by asking the individual and any bystanders what happened, when it happened, where it happened and possibly why it happened. Find out more about the injury by looking at how the incident occurred. For example, if in a Formula 1 race two cars crash into each other sideways, injuries are likely to be on the side of the body nearest to the impact. If someone has dived into the shallow end of a swimming pool and hit his head, he is likely to have a neck injury. Find out how the person is feeling. He may be able to tell you about an illness and how the illness makes him feel. The best example of this is a diabetic person who can tell you when his blood sugar is low. Find out more about the person's injuries by examining him and carrying out a head-to-toe survey (see oppposite).

key skills

Always listen to what the person tells you about his symptoms. This is especially important for people who have long-term conditions like asthma or diabetes. These people live with their condition and are often well informed about treatment.

the head-to-toe survey

A systematic head-to-toe survey is important to avoid missing vital clues about a person's injuries. Start with the head and work down the body to the toes. While you are doing the survey, think about what might be the likely problem and work with a high level of suspicion. Often it is not possible to make a definite diagnosis as many tests are only available in hospital, but it is possible to suspect an injury or illness and give the correct first-aid treatment.

how you can gain more information about the problem

Look for external clues such as objects that could have caused injury, a warning bracelet giving medical history, a card indicating diabetes, allergy or epilepsy, an inhaler that may indicate asthma and an auto injector that indicates a possibility of anaphylaxis.

then look for general signs and symptoms

Ask the person if he has pain anywhere. If the answer is yes, look at that area for injury. Check the quality of the breathing. If it is fast, slow or laboured, suspect a chest injury. Check the quality of the pulse. If it is fast, and irregular, suspect shock. Look at the skin. If there is blueness around the lips, suspect breathing problems. Feel the skin. If it is cold and clammy, suspect shock.

one-minute wonder

Q If I am assessing a person and I find that he has cold clammy skin and a fast weak pulse what should I suspect?

A Shock.

- Look around the head and neck. If you suspect a neck injury, take care not to move the head. Move your hands carefully over the person's head. Feel for blood that would indicate a scalp wound, or a depression in the skull that would indicate a skull fracture.
- Look for any blood or yellow fluid coming from the nose or the ears – this is indicative of a fracture of the skull. Look for bleeding, bruising, swelling or a foreign object in the eyes. Look at the pupils. If they are different sizes after a head injury, this indicates cerebral compression – a condition that needs early admission to hospital. Look for swelling, bleeding or bruising around the mouth and smell the person's breath – can you detect alcohol? Look at the neck for a medical-warning necklace. Feel along both collarbones for irregularity that will indicate a fracture.
- Look at the chest, the back and the abdomen. Ask the person about back pain. If there is back pain accompanied by problems moving the legs, numbness or tingling, do not allow the person to move in case there is a serious back injury that may lead to paralysis. Look at the chest for wounds.

Ask the person to take a deep breath and watch the movement. If there is unequal movement there may be a chest injury. Listen for wheezing as this may indicate asthma. Look for wounds, swelling, bruising or bleeding around the chest or abdomen. Feel the abdomen for any tenderness, bruising and muscle tightness that may indicate an internal injury. Look for incontinence – the person may have had a seizure. Feel the pelvis for deformity as this may indicate a fracture.

- Look at the limbs for any wounds, swelling, bruising, bleeding or deformity. Look for needle marks and for a medical-warning bracelet. Look at the nails for signs of blueness – this may show the person is cold.

5 5

monitoring vital signs

Having completed the primary survey to assess whether or not life-saving measures are required, and having performed the secondary survey to try to find out the problem and having given the correct first-aid treatment, you should take some baseline measurements of breathing, pulse and level of response for all injured people while waiting for the emergency services to arrive. If possible you should take these measurements regularly and record them as they can be used to monitor whether the person's condition is improving or deteriorating.

how to take the pulse

To take the pulse at the wrist, place two fingers at the base of the thumb just below the wrist creases. To take the pulse in the neck, place two fingers on the side of the person's neck between the windpipe and the large muscle in the neck.

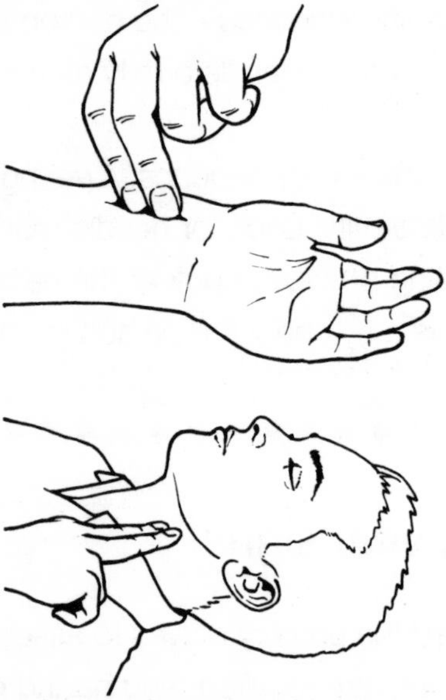

(a) By the wrist

(b) By the neck

Fig 1 Taking the pulse

Assess whether the pulse is fast or slow, weak or strong, regular or irregular. The normal rate in an average adult is between 60 and 80 beats per minute and is faster in young children – up to 120 beats per minute.

how to monitor breathing

Listen to the person's breaths and watch the chest rise and fall. Try to do this without the person realizing because we are all able to voluntarily control our breathing. Listen for wheezing or breathing difficulties.

Assess whether the breathing is fast or slow, deep or shallow, easy, difficult or painful. The normal rate in an average adult is between 12 and 16 breaths per minute and in small children can be up to 30 breaths per minute.

how to check the level of response

Ask yourself:

- Is the person alert and responding normally to your conversation? If the answer is yes the person is said to be **alert** and fully conscious.
- Is the person not fully alert but responding to voice and answering simple questions? If the answer is yes, the person is said to be responding to **voice**.
- Does the person not respond to voice but respond to pain? If the answer is yes, the person is said to respond to **pain**.
- Is the person **unresponsive** to any stimuli? If the answer is yes, the person is unconscious.

Try to remember these letters, **A**, **V**, **P**, **U**.

key skills

Baseline measurements of the person's breathing and pulse are important in confirming the diagnosis and resulting treatment, but don't forget to record them and pass them on to the ambulance crew. Remembering them will be difficult in an emergency.

one-minute wonder

Q Is it true that you can take a pulse in other places in the body apart from the wrist?

A Yes, there are pulse points in other places other than the wrist – these include the neck, the groin and the feet. The wrist is probably the easiest and most accessible place to take a pulse.

other factors to consider

When dealing with an emergency other things to watch out for include: the dangers of cross-infection, the presence of shock and the anxiety you will feel when the emergency is over.

the dangers of cross-infection

In any situation when you are dealing with other people there is a potential risk of transferring infective organisms such as viruses and bacteria from one person to another. This is especially possible when dealing with body fluids particularly blood and other body fluids contaminated with blood. Therefore it is wise to take some simple precautions. Wash your hands if possible before and after each contact and wear disposable gloves if possible. If gloves are not available do not hold back from life saving. Use the person's own hands to put pressure on a bleeding wound. If you do not have gloves you can cover your hands with clean plastic bags and cover any wounds you have on your hands with waterproof dressings. Try to avoid blood splashes in your eyes or mouth and if you are splashed in the eye, nose, mouth or in a skin wound, wash thoroughly and seek advice from your doctor. Use a plastic bag to dispose of any soiled rubbish and tie it securely around the top.

key skills

To avoid hand cross-infection when treating a person, you should wash your hands, wear gloves if they are available and cover cuts or wounds on your hands.

5

shock

Shock is a term used to describe a range of situations from feelings of anxiety to a serious clinical state in which the body has lost a lot of blood or body fluids. It is important to be aware of the difference. In all emergency situations there will be a feeling of shock and anxiety about what has happened.

This feeling will be severe amongst all involved if it is a serious incident with a lot of injured people.

Clinical shock is common after injury and is a life-threatening state in which the circulating fluid in the body is reduced and organs such as the heart and brain do not get enough blood and therefore not enough oxygen and nutrients for them to function properly. It is most commonly as a result of blood loss, but it can be caused by fluid loss as in burns.

If you suspect shock, look for the following:
- an injury or illness leading to shock
- pale, cold, clammy skin, restlessness, yawning, sighing, nausea and thirst
- a rapid and then weak pulse and fast and shallow breathing
- gradual loss of consciousness.

To help a person in shock you should treat the underlying problem if possible. Help the person to lie down and reassure him constantly as he will be very anxious. Raise the legs above the level of the heart so that the blood in the legs flows down towards the heart and the brain where it is most needed. Keep the person warm by covering with a light blanket, but remember overheating will make the shock worse because it will divert blood to the skin when it is actually needed in the vital organs such as the brain. Monitor and record the vital signs – pulse, breathing and level of response – regularly until help arrives and do not give the person anything to eat or drink as further treatment requiring an anaesthetic may be necessary in hospital.

key skills

To treat shock you should reassure the person, raise the legs and keep the person warm.

5 5

anxiety when the emergency is over

An emergency is a distressing experience for everyone involved. At the time when you are dealing with the problems you will be active and focused on what you are doing but when it is over and the emergency services have taken the people to hospital and cleared up you are likely to start asking yourself whether you did the right things, whether you phoned for help early enough, whether you got enough help from the bystanders and what will happen to the injured people.

Asking yourself these questions is completely normal and you must realize that you will feel uncertain and anxious about what happened and what you did to help. This is likely to be how everyone involved is feeling, including any medical and emergency services staff.

You may also feel angry and sad if the outcome of the emergency is poor and people have died.

It is good to talk and to help you face up to your emotions you should talk about how you feel with a friend or colleague. It would be very good to talk to someone else who was involved in the emergency so that you can share your experience. Confidentiality is important so you shouldn't talk to others about specific people involved in the emergency by name or use other personal identification but there is no reason why you can't talk about your feelings.

If you release your feelings soon after the emergency you will probably be able to cope more easily than if you keep your feelings inside you. However, you may still experience feelings of anxiety for some time after the event. You may suffer from flashbacks of what happened, nightmares or disturbed sleep, sweating and tremors, nausea – especially when thinking about what happened, tension and irritability, feelings of isolation and lack of self-confidence. If you continue to suffer from any of these problems you should ask for help from your doctor.

summary

Dealing with an emergency can be a very traumatic and occasionally distressing experience, so try and remain calm and do things in a logical manner. Try and remember the key bits of the primary and secondary surveys. Most importantly, don't forget to call for an ambulance.

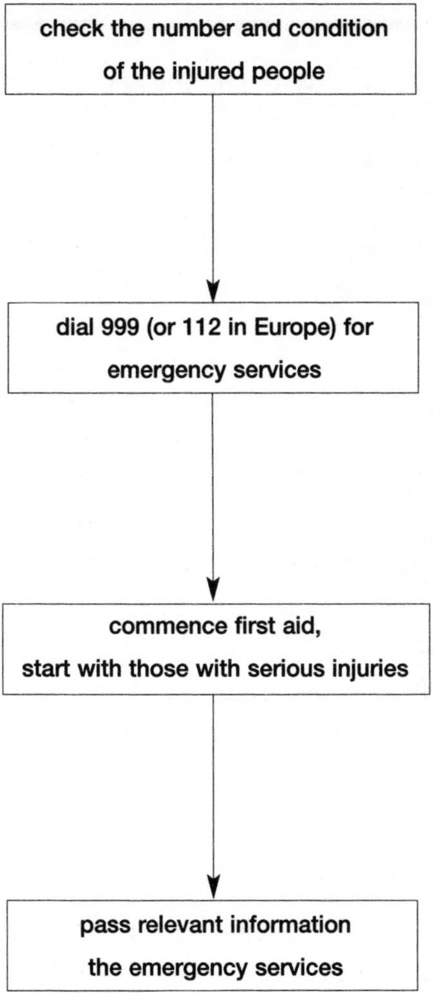

On approaching an emergency situation

self-testers

1 **Which emergency services can you access by dialing 999?**

a fire service

b gas utility service

c NHS Direct

d fell rescue service

e ambulance service

2 **Which of the following dangers will stop you from approaching an emergency?**

a toxic fumes

b swimming pool of water

c bomb blast

d moving vehicles

e falling masonry

3 **When you are monitoring a casualty's level of response what do the letters A, V, P, U stand for?**

4 **Which of the following indicate shock?**

a cold, clammy skin

b strong, slow pulse

c thirst

d slow breathing

e sighing and yawning

5 To treat shock you should:

- **a** take the person's clothes off
- **b** raise the head and shoulders
- **c** treat the underlying cause
- **d** stand the person up
- **e** raise the legs

6 Which of the following will reduce the chance of cross-infection?

- **a** washing your hands after dealing with each person
- **b** putting a waterproof dressing on the cut on your hand
- **c** avoiding splashes of blood getting in your eye
- **d** wearing disposable gloves
- **e** disposing of all soiled rubbish in a sealed plastic bag

---

answers

1 **a, d** and **e**

2 **a, c** and **e**

3 **A**lert, responds to **V**oice, responds to **P**ain, **U**nresponsive

4 **a, c** and **e**

5 **c** and **e**

6 **a**, **b**, **c**, **d** and **e**

2

how to resuscitate

Finding a person who is collapsed and needs resuscitation is a frightening experience and so it is important to try to remain calm and think clearly. You should know when to call an ambulance and be ready to give the ambulance service personnel an indication of the urgency of the situation. If the person is not breathing you will need to breathe for him. If there are no signs of heart activity you will need to do chest compressions.

In this chapter you will learn how to check for response, how to check for breathing and how to do chest compressions. You will also be advised as to the best time to call an ambulance.

how to assess an injured or ill person

When assessing a person you must first find out whether the person is conscious or unconscious – the easiest and most effective way of doing this is to check if you get a response. If the person responds to you then you will know he is conscious and therefore not in need of resuscitation.

To check response, you should talk to the person using his name if you know it and gently shake his shoulders. If you are dealing with a child aged between one and seven years old it is best not to shake but instead tap the child on the shoulder.

If there is no response, shout for someone in the vicinity to come and help you and ask yourself whether the person's airway is open.

The initial assessment of an injured person is known as the ABC of resuscitation:

- A – Airway
- B – Breathing
- C – Circulation.

These are described in detail in the following five-minute sections.

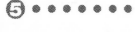

5 5

open the airway

Place one hand on the forehead of the casualty and gently tilt his head backwards. This will allow the mouth to fall open so that you will be able to see any obvious obstructions to the airway around the mouth or nose. If there is an obvious obstruction, remove it and then put the fingertips of your other hand under the point of the person's chin and lift.

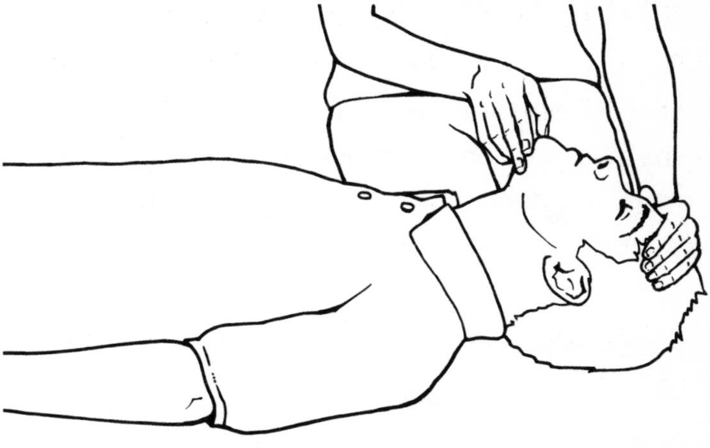

Fig 2 How to open the airway

key skills

To open the airway you should place two fingers under the person's chin and lift the chin, tilting the head back. This moves the tongue forward and opens the airway.

one-minute wonder

Q Should a gum shield always be removed?

A Yes it is best to remove a gum shield because it usually becomes dislodged and will therefore potentially block the airway and get in the way if you need to do rescue breaths.

check for breathing

With the airway open you can now check to see if the person is breathing. To check for breathing you place your head down over the mouth and nose and look along the chest to see if it is moving up and down. Listen for the sound of breathing and feel for the breath on your cheek. Do this for about ten seconds.

one-minute wonder

Q People often talk of swallowing the tongue – what does this mean?

A The tongue is not actually swallowed but when you lose consciousness you also lose muscle tone and if you are lying on your back the tongue can flop into the back of the throat and block the airway. When you tip the head back, the tongue regains its normal position in the floor of the mouth.

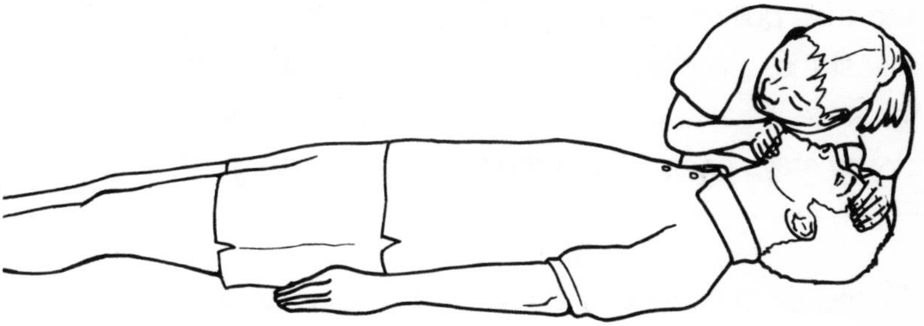

Fig 3 How to check breathing

If the person is breathing look for any other life-threatening injuries such as severe bleeding and deal with these (see Chapter 3, page 51). Then place the person in the recovery position (see below).

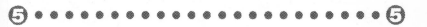

the recovery position

Kneel beside the person and remove spectacles and any bulky objects from the pocket on the side you are going to roll the person onto (the side nearest to you). Place the arm that is nearest to you at a right angle to the person's body.

Bend the elbow, and face the palm upwards. Bring the other arm across the body and hold the back of this hand against the person's cheek. With your other hand grasp the person's far leg just above the knee and pull it up until the foot is flat on the floor and then pull on the far leg and roll the person towards you. Adjust the upper leg so that it is at right angles at the hip and the knee. Finally, tilt the person's head back to make sure the airway stays open. This is the finished recovery position (see Figure 4).

The recovery position is the safest position possible for the injured person because if he is sick the vomit will drain away, the airway stays open, and the chest can move freely making breathing as good as possible and the position is stable.

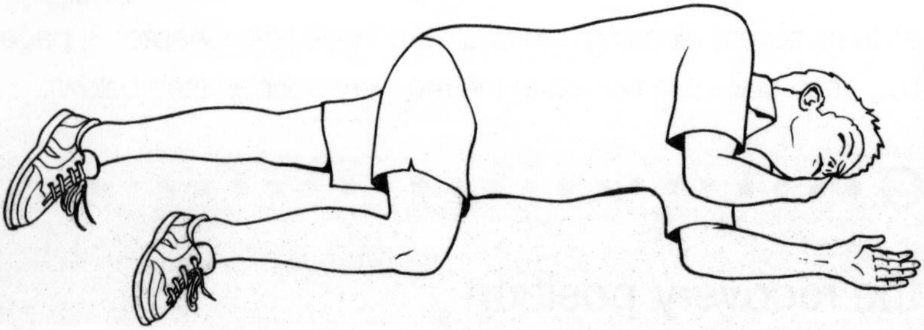

Fig 4 The finished recovery position

key skills

If a person is unconscious and breathing, whatever the cause, you should place him in the recovery position. You can then ask someone to call for an ambulance if necessary.

one-minute wonder

Q If I have to go to a telephone to get help is it safe to leave the person?

A Ideally you should send someone else to telephone for help, but if you have to do this yourself make sure you have made the person as safe as you possibly can by putting him into the recovery position.

5 • 5

rescue breaths

If the person is not breathing, call the emergency services and give two rescue breaths. To perform rescue breaths, or the 'kiss of life', keep the airway open, pinch the nose and place your mouth around the person's mouth. Blow steadily until the chest rises (see Figure 5). Then take your mouth away and watch the chest fall. If the chest rises as you blow and falls as you take your mouth away, you have given an effective breath. For an adult you should give a rescue breath every six seconds and for a child the rate is every three seconds.

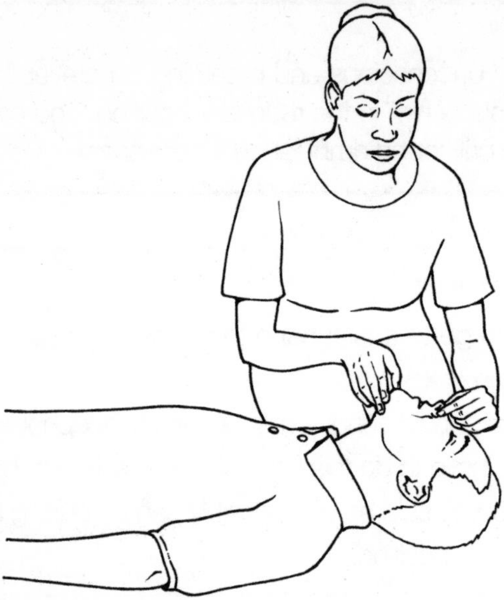

(a) Tilt the head back and pinch the nose.

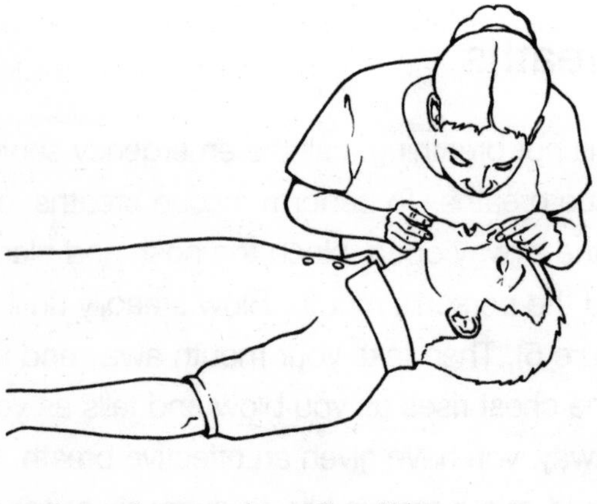

(b) Place your mouth over the person's mouth and blow.

Fig 5 How to give rescue breaths

Once you have given two effective rescue breaths you need to check for any signs of blood circulation. The signs to look for are breathing, coughing or movement of the body or limbs. Take a quick look for no longer than ten seconds. If there are no signs you should try to provide some artificial blood circulation by doing chest compressions, or 'chest pumps'. If there is circulation continue with rescue breaths.

5 • 5

chest compressions

Kneel beside the person and find the lower part of his breastbone. Do this by using your middle finger of one hand to find the point where the lowermost rib meets the breastbone. Place your index finger on the breastbone beside your middle finger, run the heel of your other hand down the breastbone and place it next to the fingers. This is the point you apply pressure. For an adult, place the heel of one hand on the breastbone, then place the heel of your other hand on top and interlock your fingers. Lean over the person and, keeping your arms straight, press down by about 4–5 cm (1.5–2 inches) at a rate of 100 compressions per minute (see Figure 6). For a child, use one hand and press down one third of the depth of the chest at the same rate as for an adult. Release the pressure without taking your hands off the chest.

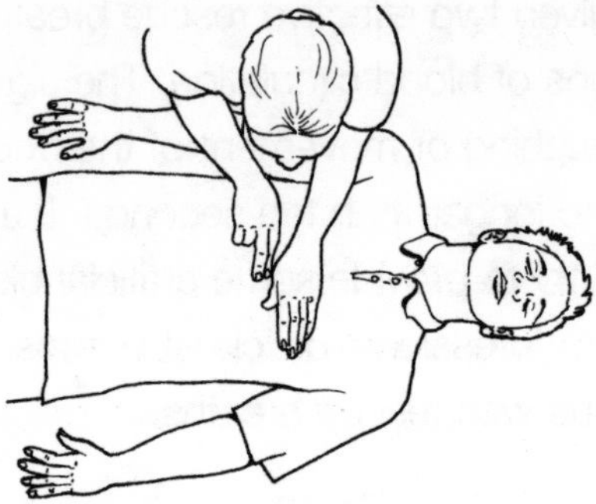

(a) Run the heel of your hand down the breastbone and place it next to your two fingers.

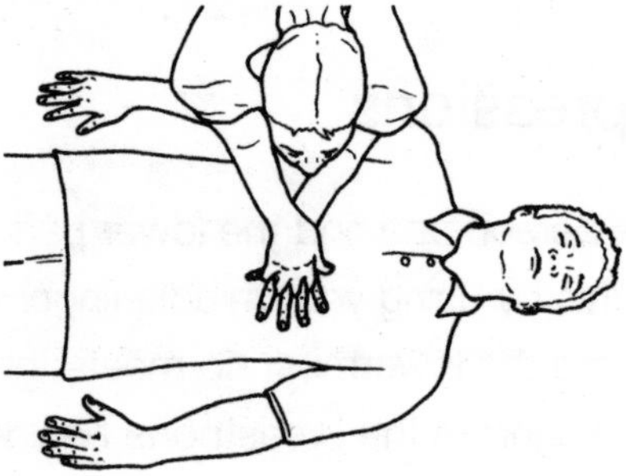

(b) Place the heel of your other hand on top and interlock your fingers.

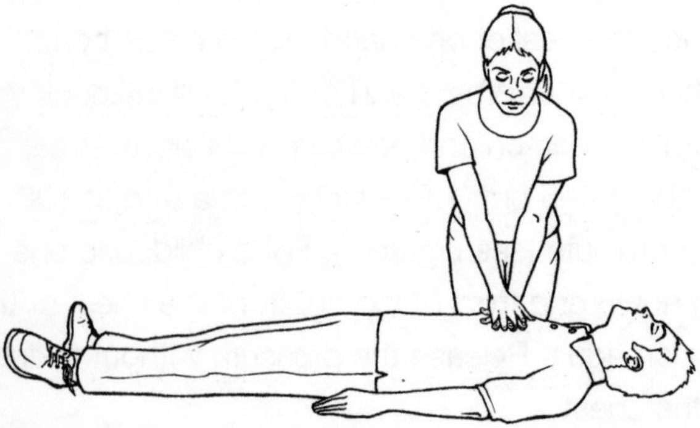

(c) Keep your arms straight and use the heel of your hands to press down.

Fig 6 How to perform chest compressions

CPR

CPR, cardio pulmonary resuscitation is the combination of chest compressions with rescue breaths at a ratio of two breaths to 15 chest compressions for an adult and one breath to five compressions for a child.

When performing CPR continue until help arrives and takes over, you are so exhausted you cannot carry on, or the person takes a breath or makes a movement. In a remote setting it is difficult to know whether to go for help or start resuscitation. You can attract attention by shouting, blowing a whistle or sending up a flare (if you have one) but if there is no prospect of being able to call for help it is probably best to start CPR and carry on for as long as you can as someone else might come along to help you. This action also gives the person the best chance of survival.

***one-minute** wonder*

Q Will I damage the heart if there is still a faint heartbeat and I do chest compressions?

A This is a very small risk but the benefits of doing chest compressions in this situation very much outweigh that risk.

one-minute wonder

Q Will I restart the heart by doing chest compressions?

A This is unlikely – to restart the heart you need a defibrillator, a machine that sends an electrical charge across the heart to try to restart it. By doing chest compressions you are maintaining some blood circulation while waiting for the emergency services to bring a defibrillator.

key skills

To perform CPR on an adult you should deliver two rescue breaths followed by 15 chest compressions. Continue until the the ambulance crew arrives and takes over from you.

the jaw thrust

There is another way of opening the airway, this is known as the jaw thrust. This is a good technique to use if you suspect an unconscious person has a neck injury as it reduces the amount of movement of the neck while at the same time opening the airway. It is of particular use in sporting injuries as the chances of a serious injury to the neck are high in activities such as rugby, motor sport and horse riding.

how to do the jaw thrust

You will need to kneel behind the person's head and place your hands on each side of his face with your fingers below the ear lobes behind the points where the lower jaw turns forwards. Then you gently lift the jaw so that it juts up into the air and this will open the airway (see Figure 7). When you do this you must take care that you don't tilt the neck. If you then need to check breathing you will have to lean forward to listen for breathing and feel it on your cheek.

If the person is breathing and there is no sign that he is going to vomit then you can keep the airway open by staying in this position. If, however, you have difficulty using the jaw thrust to keep the airway open or you have to leave the person to dial for an ambulance or you have to give rescue breaths, you should revert to the head tilt–chin lift technique as described on page 29.

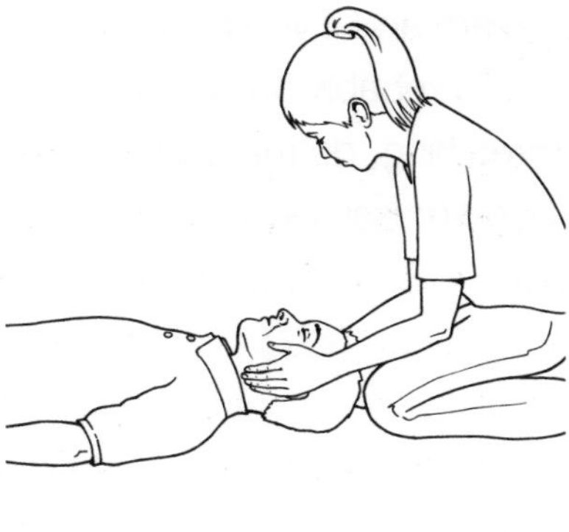

Fig 7 The jaw thrust technique

one-minute wonder

Q Which takes priority – life saving or taking care of the neck?

A While care of the neck is very important as further damage may lead to paralysis, life saving must always take priority.

one-minute wonder

Q How do I know where the angle of the jaw is?

A If you feel down from the ear lobes on either side you will feel the jaw comes straight down and then bends forwards towards chin. The angle is the point of the bend.

summary

CPR is probably one of the best known but least understood first-aid procedures. It is the single most important life-saving technique you can learn and if you have to carry out CPR, our research tells us it will probably be on a person known to you. If the person is not breathing, do rescue breaths; if the heart is not working, do chest compressions.

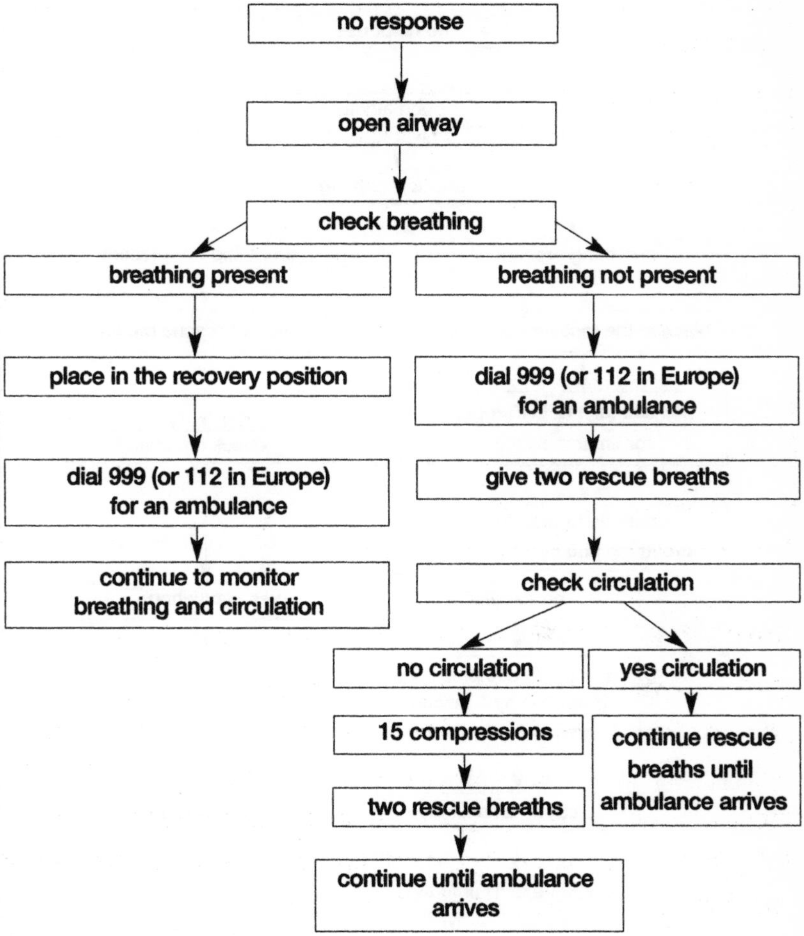
no response
open airway
check breathing
breathing present
breathing not present
place in the recovery position
dial 999 (or 112 in Europe) for an ambulance
continue to monitor breathing and circulation
dial 999 (or 112 in Europe) for an ambulance
give two rescue breaths
check circulation
no circulation
yes circulation
15 compressions
two rescue breaths
continue until ambulance arrives
continue rescue breaths until ambulance arrives

How to respond to an unconscious adult

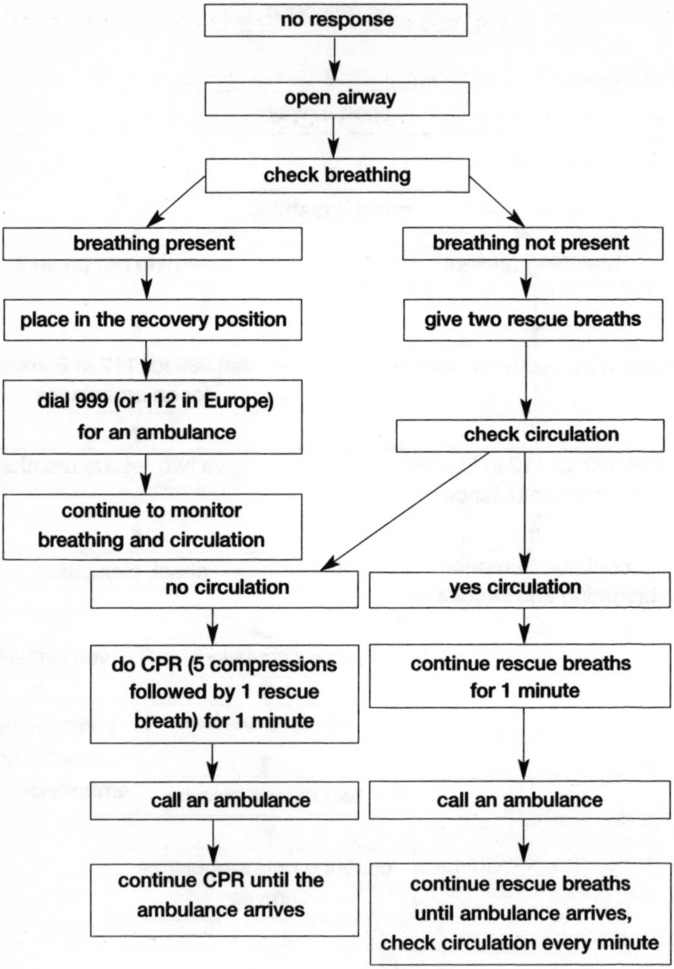
no response
open airway
check breathing
breathing present
place in the recovery position
dial 999 (or 112 in Europe) for an ambulance
continue to monitor breathing and circulation
breathing not present
give two rescue breaths
check circulation
no circulation
do CPR (5 compressions followed by 1 rescue breath) for 1 minute
call an ambulance
continue CPR until the ambulance arrives
yes circulation
continue rescue breaths for 1 minute
call an ambulance
continue rescue breaths until ambulance arrives, check circulation every minute

How to respond to an unconscious child (aged one to seven years inclusive)

self-testers

1 The recovery position is a safe position because:

a if the person is sick the vomit will drain away

b the airway stays open

c the tongue doesn't drop back into the throat

d the chest can move freely

e it is a stable position

2 When checking for a response in a child you should:

a shake the child

b hold the child upside down

c tap the child's shoulder

d speak loudly and clearly

e slap the child between the shoulder blades

3 When doing rescue breathing for an adult, the rate is:

a every three seconds

b every 10 seconds

c every 20 seconds

d every six seconds

e every 15 seconds

4 When checking for signs of circulation you should look for:

a moving

b eye opening

c breathing

d coughing

e colour of the skin

5 The ratio for rescue breaths to chest compressions for an adult is:

a 2:15
b 1:5
c 3:12
d 5:50
e 2:10

6 The rate for chest compressions:

a varies for adults and children
b is 100 per minute for all ages
c depends on the size of the person
d is 80 per minute for all ages
e depends on how fast you can do them

answers

1 **a, b, c, d** and **e**
2 **c** and **d**
3 **d**
4 **a, b, c** and **d**
5 **a**
6 **b**

5 minute first aid

3

in the gym

A significant number of injuries that occur in the gym are the result of not warming up and cooling down properly. Others result from not using the equipment in the way it was designed. Injuries also occur because people over-estimate their strength and level of fitness. Some freak accidents also occur in the gym – members dropping dumb-bells on their toes or on the feet of another gym user are not as uncommon as we might think.

Here are some of the things you may wish to consider before using equipment.

Firstly, have you gone through a proper warm up routine? Most gym users have their own preferred way of warming up, if you need advice, the gym instructors will be able to help. Then, look around the area you are exercising in. Will your exercises impact on anyone else using the area? If so, ensure there is sufficient room between you and the other gym users. If someone else is exercising close by, let him know the type of exercises you intend to do so he is aware of your presence.

Most gym equipment is mechanical in the way it operates. Some of the equipment involves the movement of heavy loads, not just once but a number of times; this may result in you becoming fatigued. The combination of these things means you should exercise with caution when using the equipment.

Look at the equipment before using it, does it look safe, has it been modified in any way by a previous user that may present a danger to you? Are the handgrips secure and the cables moving as they should? If you have used the equipment before does it feel as you think it should feel? If not, consult the staff before using it.

5 5

crush injuries

Moving weights and operating gym equipment inevitably means that injuries, both minor and more serious, can occur. Crushed and trapped fingers and toes (digits) are among the more common types of injuries found in the gym.

Trapped fingers and toes can be extremely painful and, to reduce the pain and long-term damage associated with this type of injury, it is important to release the digits as quickly as possible. Once the digits have been released, you should inspect the site of the injury. This type of injury can result in a wound or bone injury or, in more serious cases, a combination of the two.

If there is a loss of blood and you suspect there may be some underlying damage to the bones, you should apply a clean pad to the injured area. All gyms should have a stock of first-aid supplies, so getting access to a clean, non-fluffy pad should not be too difficult. The fingers and toes do not have a large amount of tissue surrounding them so in some crush injuries you may be able to see the bone. In injuries like this, it is important to keep the flesh and bone as clean as possible, which is why it is preferable to use a clean, sterile pad, if possible, sterile pad.

Avoid applying too much pressure to the injured area and don't ask the injured person to try and move their digits as part of your assessment of the injury. This will only increase the pain with the more serious injuries and will not give you any vital information.

Many of us forget the most obvious things in emergency situations like this. One of the more important things you should do is get the person to sit down. Assuming that the person is sitting down with a clean or sterile pad in place, you should then elevate the injured area. Your aim should be to keep the hand or foot above the level of the heart.

Once the area is elevated, you can apply some ice to help reduce the swelling and control further blood loss. Do not apply ice directly to the skin as it can cause a cold burn. Place the ice in a plastic bag or wrap it in a cloth or towel and place this on the affected area.

one-minute wonder

Q You mention that you should apply a clean pad to the injured area. Can you use cotton wool?

A Avoid cotton wool if you can as it tends to stick to the wound and when the person is treated in hospital, the cotton wool will have to be removed, causing more pain or discomfort.

In crush injuries where there is no break in the skin or there is no obvious bone damage, you may see the fingernails or the toenails turn blue, which is a result of blood gettiing trapped under the nail. This often results in a throbbing pain. Applying ice can often help but the injured person may have to go to hospital for a minor procedure to release the trapped blood.

key skills

To treat a trapped digit:

- release the trapped digit
- treat any bleeding by applying a clean pad
- elevate the area
- apply ice
- seek medical advice or arrange for the person to be taken to hospital.

one-minute wonder

Q I read in a magazine that if a person is crushed for more than 15 minutes you should not release him. Is this correct?

A Yes. If you know the person has been trapped for more than 15 minutes, you should not release him. Call for the emergency services as soon as possible and wait for them to arrive.

Crush injuries to large parts of the body, such as the leg or chest, where the person remains trapped for longer than 15 minutes, can result in a build up of toxins, which can be dangerous if released. In this situation you should not release the person but call the emergency services. In the most serious crush injuries the toxins will spread around the body and can permanently damage key organs including the kidneys and so resist your instinct to try to release the person. This is a difficult thing to do especially if the person is in pain.

5 5

severe bleeding

Blood loss from the body can occur in two main ways – internal and external bleeding. In internal bleeding the blood is actually lost from the circulation, but leaks into another part of the body.

It can occur for a number of reasons but in terms of sporting activities it will most likely result from a violent blow to the body, possibly the abdomen. If you suspect the person may have internal bleeding you should first inspect the site of the injury. Are there any signs of bruising, swelling or tenderness? The person may also have a fast and weak pulse, his breathing may be fast, he will look pale and his skin may be be cold to the touch. Bleeding from the nose, mouth, ear, anus, urethra and vagina may also indicate internal injury. If inspecting these areas for blood loss, ensure you advise the person and maintain his dignity. The person may also begin to show signs of shock (see Chapter 1, page 20).

To treat a person with suspected internal bleeding, you should treat as for shock (see Chapter 1, page 20).

key skills

Internal bleeding can be difficult to diagnose in a first-aid setting. Consider the mechanics of the injury and treat for shock. If necessary, call for an ambulance.

External bleeding is much easier to diagnose than internal bleeding as it is visible. In severe bleeding there is damage to the underlying blood vessels, including the veins and arteries. There are various types of wounds including incisions, lacerations and puncture wounds.

When treating a large wound your aim as a first aider is to control the bleeding, reduce the chances of the wound becoming infected and prevent the person going into shock. When dealing with any body fluids, including blood, you should take some basic infection-control procedures like wearing disposable rubber gloves.

how to treat severe bleeding

The first thing you should do when treating a severe bleed is to take a quick look at the wound to make sure there is nothing embedded in it. You should then apply direct pressure over the wound using your hand. If the person is capable of doing this, you should ask him to do it. Once pressure has been applied, you should then raise the limb above the level of the heart. If the injury is to the person's leg, you should lay him down first and then raise the leg. This will reduce blood supply to the injured area. You should then place a clean, pad or any clean, non-fluffy material like a towel over the wound and ensure pressure is maintained. Of course, if you have a first-aid kit available, you can use the correct size dressing to bandage the wound. If treating an arm injury, you should also lay the person down to safeguard against the possibility of him going into shock.

key skills

When treating severe bleeding:

- apply direct pressure to the wound
- elevate the affected area
- apply a dressing
- call for an ambulance.

one-minute wonder

Q You say the wound should be checked first to see if there is anything embedded in it. How should I treat the blood loss if there is something stuck in the wound?

A Do not remove any object like a piece of glass as this may be stopping some blood escaping and you may do more damage if you attempt to remove it. In this case you should apply pressure to the edges of the wound and bandage around and over the wound without applying direct pressure to the embedded object.

amputation

A finger, toe or in some cases a limb that becomes completely amputated needs specific first-aid care. The advances in surgery mean that in many cases the severed digit or limb can be re-attached by microsurgery. Whether this is achievable or not is partly dependent on what you, the first aider, do with the severed part of the body.

In this situation, you should remember that your priority is to treat the injured person rather than care for the severed part. When amputations occur as a result of an accident, there is often significant blood loss and you must treat the bleeding. You must apply direct pressure to the wound and elevate it above the level of the heart. You should also be aware of the risk of the person going into shock. To treat shock, lay the person down, elevate the legs and cover the person with a blanket to keep him warm. Do not give the person anything to eat or drink because he is likely to need a general anaesthetic in hospital.

With an amputation, you should try and prevent the condition of the amputated part deteriorating. It is important to keep the body part as clean as possible but do not wash it. If gloves are available you should handle the part with these and place it in a plastic bag or wrap it in cling film. Then immediately wrap the bag in some soft fabric material and place it in a container of ice. It is important that the severed part does not come into direct contact with the ice. Label the container with the time of injury and the person's name and ensure it goes to hospital with the injured person.

key skills

In the event of an amputation of a body part, you should care for the person's injury first. Then place the amputated part in a plastic bag or wrap with cling film and place in a container of ice. Send the part to hospital with the injured person.

one-minute wonder

Q If a person's ear is cut and bleeding, how do I stop the bleeding as the wound is already above the level of the heart?

A As the wound is already elevated, sit the person down and apply direct pressure to the wound. If the ear is severed, care for it as described above for a toe or finger.

summary

Some gym injuries can be avoided and others occur as a result of overexertion or incorrect use of the equipment. Some of the injuries and treatment you should give are covered in Chapter 5.

Some gym injuries result in blood loss and possible shock. To treat severe blood loss, you should apply direct pressure and elevate. If there is an object embedded in the wound bandage around it. Remember to reassure the person while treating him. Minor cuts and grazes can be cleaned and a plaster applied.

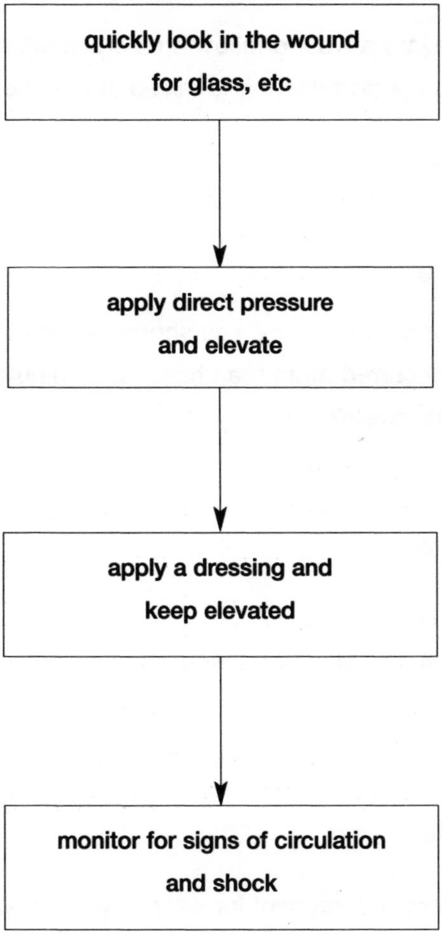

How to treat a severe bleed

self-testers

1 **When we elevate a wound following a crush injury, it will be effective and comfortable if it is raised above the person's:**

a head

b heart

c waist

d stomach

2 **In the case of a crush injury, you should not release the person if the injury occurred more than how many minutes before you arrived on the scene?**

a 15 minutes

b 5 minutes

c 20 minutes

d 35 minutes

3 **An amputated part should be wrapped and put in:**

a ice

b cold water

c milk

d warm water

4 **The most effective treatment for severe bleeding is to:**

a apply direct pressure and reassure

b elevate and reassure

c apply direct pressure, elevate and reassure

d apply direct pressure and call for an ambulance

answers

1 **b**

2 **a**

3 **a**

4 **c**

4

in the water

Water sports such as swimming, diving, snorkelling, scuba diving, sailing, windsurfing and water skiing attract large numbers of participants.

All forms of water sports present a hazard, however, the risks can be reduced if you take some very simple precautions. Both swimming pools and open water, such as fresh water, lakes, rivers and lagoons can present hazards to participants.

diving accidents

Diving is a stressful sport. A depth change of 7 m produces changes in the body equal to a trip from sea level to the top of Mount Everest.

There are many health reasons for not diving. These include:

- heart disease
- pregnancy
- perforated eardrum
- epilepsy
- diabetes
- migraine
- lung disease
- ear infection.

how to recognize diving complications

Complications of diving include:

- hypothermia
- drowning
- marine bites or stings
- decompression sickness.

To prevent diving accidents, first of all make sure you are a good swimmer. Avoid dehydration, and do the deepest part of the dive first. Time the ascent, keep warm, and make a safety stop at 4.5 m. After the dive, move around to help nitrogen removal from the blood.

decompression sickness

Decompression sickness is an emergency requiring quick transfer to a recompression chamber. It usually results from ascending too quickly from a dive.

how to recognize decompression sickness

The signs of decompression sickness are:

- vomiting
- throbbing muscle pains
- mottled skin rash
- headache
- seizures.

drowning

If water enters the mouth and nose in any significant quantity it can impact on the person's ability to breathe. Your aim in a drowning situation is to remove the person from the water as quickly as possible. It is important to carry the person with the head lower than the chest. This helps to drain the water from the airway and avoids it entering the lungs.

Once you have got the person onto dry land or to the poolside, lay him on his back. Check the airway and check if he is breathing. If he is breathing, place him in the recovery position (see Chapter 2). If he is not breathing, give rescue breaths and check circulation. If there are no signs of circulation, give chest compressions (see Chapter 2). Make sure someone has called for an ambulance. Continue CPR.

one-minute wonder

Q Is it true that you should not eat before swimming?

A Yes, swimming on a full stomach is not advised. It can result in stomach cramps and reduce your ability to swim.

key skills

If you find yourself at the scene of a drowning incident:

- get the person out of water as quickly as possible
- do not attempt any detailed assessment of his condition whilst the person is still in the water
- assess the ABC
- treat for hypothermia
- seek medical advice.

It is important to remember that you should seek medical advice even if the person appears to make a full recovery. Some near-drowning victims suffer from a condition known as 'secondary drowning', where water enters the lungs but the effects are not obvious for a number of hours.

5

hypothermia

When you remove a person from water there is a risk he will be suffering from hypothermia. To treat for hypothermia, you should remove any wet clothing, cover the person with a blanket or any dry clothing that is available. If the person is conscious, give him something warm to drink or some high-energy food like chocolate to eat (see also Chapter 6, pages 88 and 89).

***one-minute** wonder*

Q You say put a dry blanket over a person. I was told that if you only have one blanket, you should put it under the person, as he will retain more heat that way.

A Ideally, you should have a blanket or clothing over and under the person. It is true that by lying on cold or wet ground, a person can lose a lot of heat. If you do not have enough clothing and you are outside, lie the person on thick undergrowth or vegetation.

***one-minute** wonder*

Q Is it dangerous to give a person suffering from hypothermia alcohol to warm him up?

A It can be. There are no medical benefits associated with giving alcohol, in fact there is evidence that it may make the condition worse.

leptospirosis

This condition, which is also known as Weils Disease, is a hazard for people who undertake water sports in lakes and rivers and any other inland water especially if the water is stagnant. This infection is usually caused by rats and other rodents and can easily transfer to humans, especially if you have an open cut or wound. Simple precautions like covering cuts and wounds before entering the water and showering afterwards can help protect against this risk. You should remember that infection might not be obvious for 7–10 days after contact. The symptoms of leptospirosis include nausea, vomiting and headaches. Some people also experience flu-like symptoms.

If you suspect you have the condition, you should seek medical advice as soon as possible.

one-minute wonder

Q Is it possible to perform CPR in water?

A It is possible to perform a modified version of CPR in water, but we know that chest compressions in particular are much more effective if delivered on a firm surface.

summary

You should treat water with respect. If in doubt about the suitability of water for your sport you should seek advice, obey signs and speak to local community members.

If you see someone getting into difficulty in water, remove him from the water as quickly as possible, then assess the person on dry land and call the emergency services if necessary. Remember, lifeguards or on occasions lifeboats may be able to give you assistance.

self-testers

1 In a drowning situation, when carrying a person you should ensure:

- **a** he is completely flat
- **b** his head is lower than his chest
- **c** his head is higher than his chest
- **d** he is in the recovery position

2 When treating someone suffering from hypothermia which of the following should you give the person to eat or drink?

- **a** alcohol
- **b** chocolate
- **c** warm drink
- **d** hot drink

3 To help protect yourself from leptospirosis you should:

a cover any open wounds with waterproof plasters

b bandage any wounds before entering water

c neither of the above

d avoid swimming in unfamiliar water

answers

1 **b**

2 **b** and **c**

3 **a** and **d**

5

on the sports field

Most sports played on fields, courts or the track present the participant with the risk of injury. Contact sports like rugby, football and hockey are more often associated with injury than non-contact sports like athletics. Even the less physically demanding sports like bowling result in a significant number of injuries including back strain.

Again, some simple precautions can help reduce the number or seriousness of the injuries. You should carry out a proper warm up and cool down and wear the recommended protective equipment. If you are playing sport for a long period or in hot weather, remember to wear sunscreen and re-hydrate regularly.

Most sporting activities including running, walking, jumping, throwing and pushing put demand on the body. Most people carry out sporting activities for enjoyment or to maintain a good physical fitness. However, some people undertake physical exercise without being in the necessary physical condition.

We know that this often happens on holiday when 'out of condition' people start playing sports they are not familiar with. This is when a large number of sports-related injuries occur.

sprains and strains

Damage to the muscle, tendons or ligaments are the most common injuries associated with playing sport. They are often referred to as 'soft-tissue injuries' by medical personnel. A sprain is an injury to the ligaments around a joint. We talk about strains in relation to muscles and tendons. The ability to differentiate between the two is not overly important, as the treatment is similar. However, the actual location of the injury will often indicate whether it is a sprain or strain. In the more popular sports like football, sprains tend to occur in the ankle and knee areas and strains in the calf and thigh. Sprains usually result from overstretching, possibly to reach a ball or to tackle an opponent. This results in the stretching of a ligament (this is the supporting structure around a joint).

The treatment for a sprain or strain is known as the **RICE** procedure.

- **R**est It is important to stop moving as soon as possible after the injury. It is only possible to 'walk off' the most minor of soft-tissue injuries. We now know that rest is key to recovery following a strain or a sprain. Applying unnecessary pressure and moving the injured part only delays the healing process. So encourage the person to sit down and take the pressure off the injured area until further treatment can be applied.
- **I**ce Applying ice to the injured part reduces the blood flow to the injury. This means that the amount of swelling and bruising is also reduced. If you do not have ice to hand use frozen vegetables. It is important you do not apply these directly to the skin as you may end up with a cold burn. Wrap the ice or vegetables in a towel or anything that will ensure a barrier between the ice and the skin. There is medical evidence to suggest that ice applied as quickly as possible to the affected area can prevent swelling and significantly speed up healing.
- **C**ompress To ensure the injured part of the body is supported apply a bandage or use one of the various support devices that are available for this purpose. If you are applying a bandage it is important that it is sufficiently tight to give support, but not too tight that it cuts off the blood supply.
- **E**levate Keep the injured part of the body above the level of the heart. This helps to reduce the swelling and aids the healing process. If the injury occurs to the arm or hand, it is important to follow exactly the same procedure. Elevation of the arm or wrist can be achieved by placing the arm in a sling as shown in Figure 8.

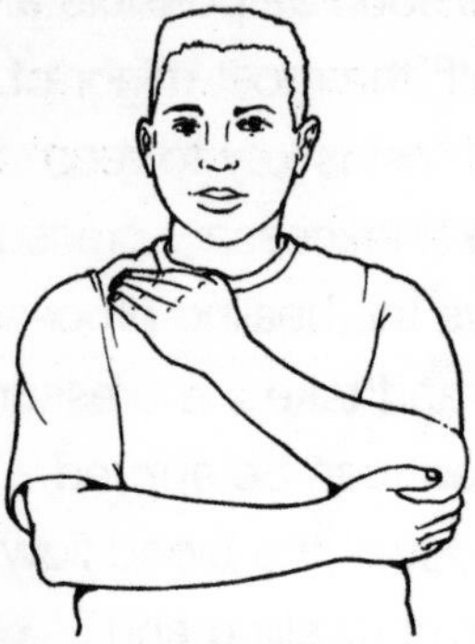

(a) Elevate the arm and support it at the elbow.

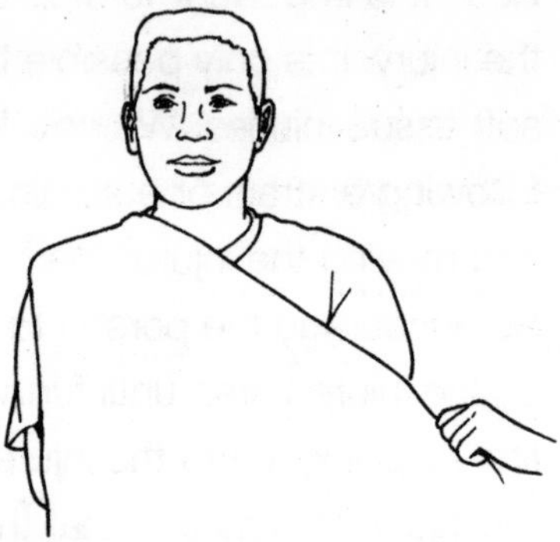

(b) Drape the triangular bandage over the uninjured shoulder.

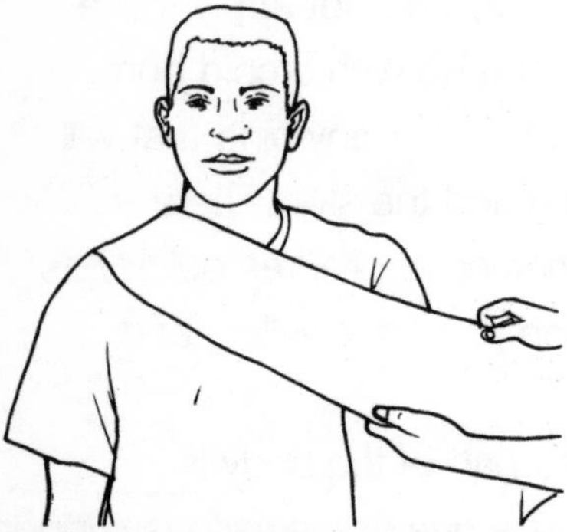

(c) The person should now release his elbow and you should tuck the base of the bandage under his injured arm.

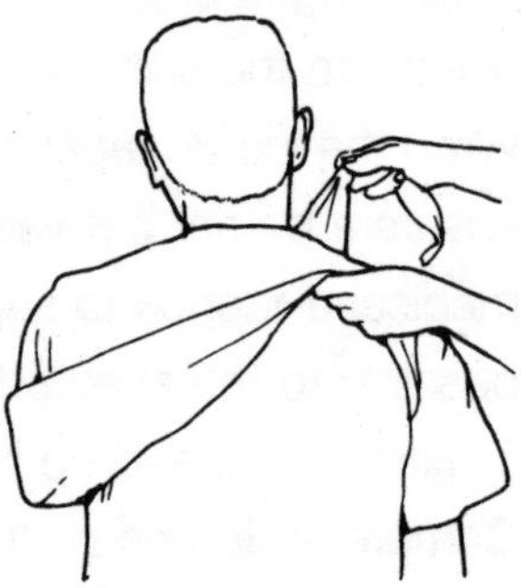

(d) Bring the lower end of the bandage across the back and tie it at the shoulder.

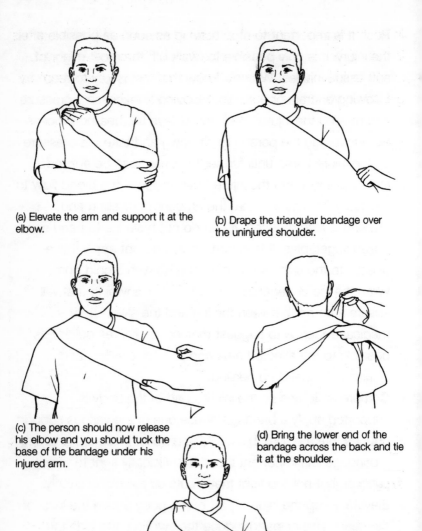

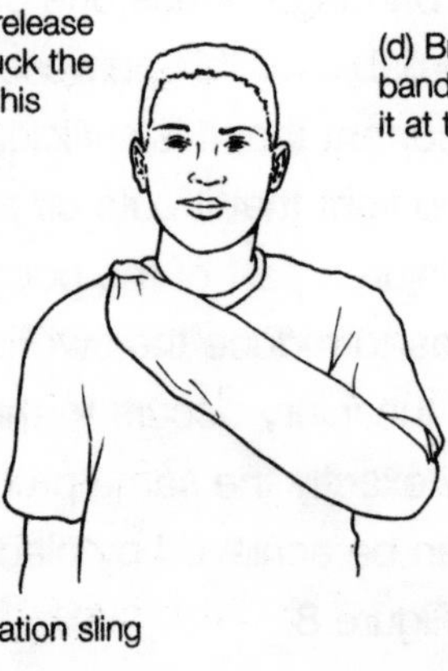

(e) Secure all loose fabric by twisting and tucking in at the elbow.

Fig 8 How to apply an elevation sling

In addition to the treatment described previously, if the person is in pain, then painkillers should be taken. There is a wide variety available in both tablet form and also in the form of a cream or gel. If the symptoms persist, get medical advice.

key skills

To treat a strain or sprain, you should remember the RICE procedure: Rest, Ice, Compress and Elevate.

one-minute wonder

Q Is it true that if a person gets a sprained ankle while playing football, you should leave the football boot on to give the ankle support?

A No, if you know that the ankle injury is a sprain and not something else, you should remove the boot, as you need to inspect the site of the injury and apply ice.

5 5

fractures

This is the term we use to describe a break in the bone. There are two main types of fracture: an open fracture and a closed fracture. In a closed fracture, the skin around the site of the fracture is not broken. In the case of an open fracture, there is a wound or break in the skin and the bone is sometimes seen.

Fractures in sports often result from contact between two players, but they can also happen if a person falls awkwardly or collides with a goalpost.

If you suspect a player has a fracture, try to find out as much as possible about the accident to give you as many clues as possible. It is also important to discover as much as you can about how the person is feeling. You can also identify a fracture by looking at the injured site as the limb may seem deformed or in an unnatural position. The person will be in obvious pain and this will increase if you attempt to move him. In some cases, you may be able to hear the grating of the bone and in the case of an open fracture there will be a break in the skin. You may also notice a shortening of the limb.

how to treat a fracture

If possible avoid moving a person with a fracture, especially if the fracture is in the leg. You should remember that fractured bones are very sharp and any unnecessary movement may result in damage to the blood vessels or organs surrounding the fracture. Your aim as a first aider is to get the person to the hospital. Call for an ambulance. Keep talking to the person and support the injury in a way that's most comfortable for him. Do not allow the person to drink or eat in case he has to have an anaesthetic in hospital.

If there is a delay in getting the person to hospital for whatever reason, you should bandage the injured part of the body to an uninjured part. For example, if the leg is fractured, the good one can be bandaged to the bad one.

key skills

If you suspect a fracture you should reassure the person, call an ambulance, discourage the person from moving and support the injury in a comfortable position until the ambulance arrives.

one-minute wonder

Q Is it true that you can hear the bone crack when there is a fracture?

A It is possible, but not always the case. But it is important to ask the injured person what he heard and felt at the time the injury was sustained.

one-minute wonder

Q What is meant by a 'clean break' when people talk about a fracture?

A People use this term to describe a break or a crack in the bone where there are two 'clean ends' with no other fragments of the bone present. This is also known as a closed fracture.

open fractures

In the case of an open fracture, where there is a wound and the bone may be exposed, it is important you cover the wound to reduce any blood loss and keep the bone ends clean. Apply a clean pad but do not press on the ends of the bone, then bandage the pad in place. If the fracture is in the leg, you should not attempt to elevate the injured leg to reduce the blood loss. Once the bandage has been applied, check the blood circulation beyond the bandage by pressing on the nail bed. The colour of the nail bed should disappear when you press and return within a few seconds. If the colour does not return, undo the bandage immediately and re-apply less tightly.

collarbone fractures

Horse riders and cyclists are among those who are most susceptible to this type of injury. It often results from putting their arms out to protect them when falling. This directs the force up the arm, putting pressure on the collarbone that runs between the shoulder blade and the top of the breastbone.

Once again, the nature of the accident may indicate whether the collarbone is damaged or not. The person may also be in severe pain with swelling in the shoulder area.

In the case of a fractured collarbone, the injured person usually knows the position in which to hold the arm to make it most comfortable. This usually means supporting the elbow with the head tilting towards the injured shoulder. Then apply an elevation sling to ensure the injury is supported (see Figure 9).

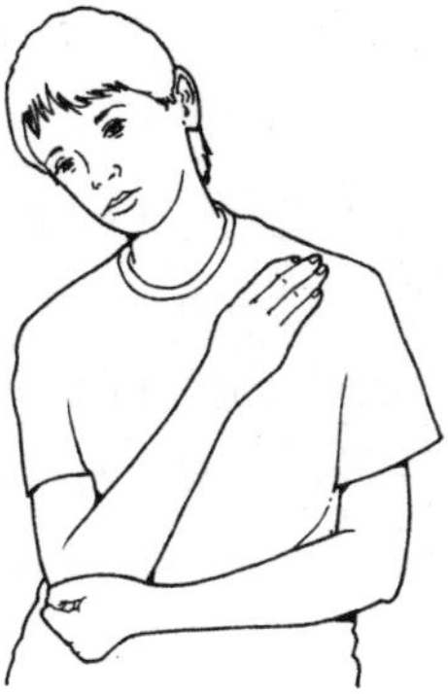

(a) Lay the affected arm across the chest diagonally with the fingertips resting against the opposite shoulder. Then apply an elevation sling.

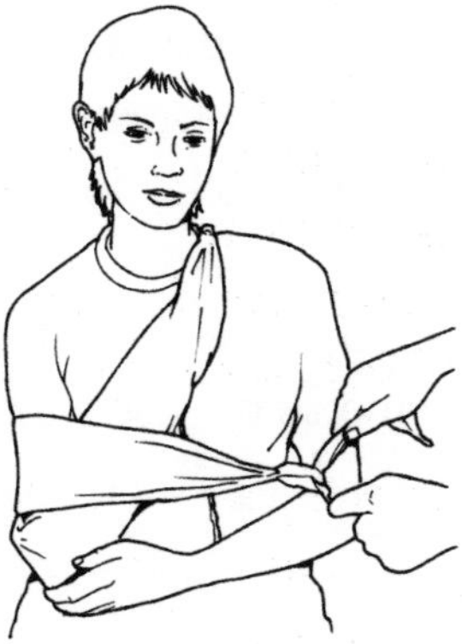

(a) Tie a bandage around the chest and over the sling to support the arm.

Fig 9 How to treat a fractured collarbone

You should then arrange for the person to be taken to hospital. It is not recommended that you lay the person down as this may increase the amount of pain, instead sit them upright.

dislocation

This type of injury occurs at the joint when the bone is pulled or twisted out of position. Dislocation most commonly occurs in the shoulder, but it can also happen to the jaw. Sports people have also been known to dislocate their fingers and thumbs. Your aim as a first aider is to stop unnecessary movement at the site of the injury.

People who have suffered a dislocation report that the pain is excruciating. You may also notice some swelling at the site of the injury. The joint may not appear normal and can be shorter than it previously was. Under no circumstances should the first aider attempt to pull the joint back into place. This is a medical procedure and should only be carried out in hospital. Encourage the injured person to support the site of the injury and, if the shoulder is involved, immobilize it using a sling and bandages as shown in Figure 10.

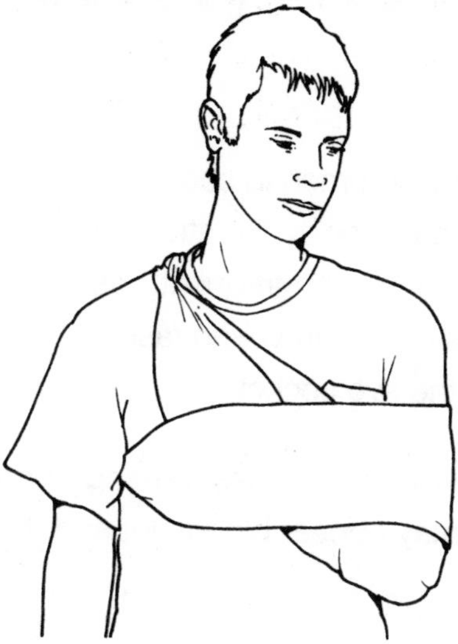

Fig 10 Use a sling to immobilize a dislocated shoulder

***one-minute** wonder*

Q Is it true that dislocated joints pop back into place if you leave them long enough?

A Some joints do not return to their natural positions without medical help, but if the joint appears to have popped back into place you should still get it checked out in hospital to confirm that it has returned to the correct position.

eye injuries

Eye injuries are very common in sport, either as a result of being hit by equipment, a ball or by the stray fist or elbow of an opponent. Squash is a sport frequently associated with eye injury as the ball is usually travelling fast and is approximately the same size as the eye socket.

Evidence of an eye injury includes swelling or bruising around the eye. The eye may appear bloodshot and the injured person may have difficulty seeing out of the injured eye.

If an eye injury occurs, get the person to sit down and put a clean pad over the eye. Ask the person to keep eye movement to a minimum. Arrange for the person to be taken to hospital. Remember, a serious injury to the eye may also indicate the possibility of a fracture to the eye socket or other facial fractures.

key skills

Eye injuries are best treated by covering the eye and taking the person to hospital.

one-minute wonder

Q What should I do if someone has a tooth knocked out?

A If a tooth becomes displaced you should attempt to put it back into its socket. If this is not possible, keep it clean and store it in milk if available. Seek dental advice.

5 • 5

head injuries

Any blow to the head that is heavy enough to cause a bruise or scalp wound can fracture the skull and lead to problems with the underlying brain such as concussion or compression. Such blows can result from a fall, contact with another person, being hit by a ball or piece of equipment or through deliberate foul play.

Concussion occurs as a result of the brain 'shaking' inside the skull. It causes a transient problem with consciousness for a few minutes but this is followed by a complete recovery. It is advisable for the person to stop playing the sport after suffering concussion in case there is a further problem, and generally the advice is that he should not restart until a medical assessment has been carried out. The rules for how long he should not play vary from sport to sport depending on the amount of physical contact associated with the sport.

Compression is less commonly associated with sport but much more serious. Bleeding inside the skull or swelling of the injured part of the brain both lead to pressure on the brain inside the skull. It is a life-threatening condition that needs immediate admission to hospital and it is important to be aware that compression may develop straight after the head injury, a few hours later or several days after the injury.

recognizing concussion

There will be a short period of impaired consciousness – anything from feeling dazed to loss of consciousness and loss of memory.

action to take

Help the person to rest. Watch for a complete recovery by looking for any change in responsiveness using the AVPU scale (see below). When the person has recovered ensure someone responsible stays with him for the next few hours and do not allow him to go back to playing sport without first getting medical advice. Advise the person to seek medical help if later he starts to suffer from a prolonged headache, vomiting, double vision or excessive drowsiness.

key skills

If a person has concussion, get him to rest. Monitor his AVPU. If the person recovers, stay with him for a few hours. Seek medical advice if the person has nausea, headaches or becomes drowsy.

the AVPU scale

The AVPU scale is used for monitoring changes in responsiveness:

- **A** Is the person fully **alert** and behaving normally?
- **V** Is the person responding to your **voice** and able to answer simple questions and obey simple commands?
- **P** Does the person open the eyes if pinched, i.e. responds to **pain**?
- **U** Is the person **unresponsive** to stimulus?

recognizing compression

The main feature of compression is a worsening level of response over time. There will also be a severe headache, a flushed face, noisy breathing and possibly a change in behaviour. If you look into the eyes you may see that the pupils are not equal in size. If the person loses consciousness check for signs of breathing.

action to take

Immediately call for an ambulance, as hospital treatment is essential. Monitor the level of response using the AVPU scale while you are waiting for the ambulance.

spinal injuries

Injuries to the spine happen in sport especially in rugby, gymnastics, trampolining, motor sports and horse riding. Damage to the spinal cord, especially in the neck, is life-changing because it can lead to paralysis of the arms and legs and is followed by a prolonged struggle to regain some movement.

recognizing a spinal injury

Always suspect a spinal injury when a person has fallen awkwardly, especially in a rugby scrum or when thrown from a horse or moving vehicle. There may be back pain, loss of feeling in the legs, inability to move the legs and, if the injury is in the neck, inability to move both the arms and legs or loss of feeling in the arms as well as the legs.

one-minute wonder

Q Will there always be loss of feeling in the legs if there is damage to the spinal cord?

A Not necessarily and this is why you must suspect damage. Always have a high level of suspicion when a person has fallen awkwardly or been thrown a distance.

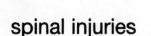

action to take

Keep the person still and call for an ambulance. Stop the sporting event and do not move the person. Support the head, neck and shoulders by using your hands to steady the head and place rolled up coats, towels or sports shirts around the neck.

If the person is unconscious do not move him. Kneel behind the person's head and support the head in line with the spine. If necessary, open the airway using the jaw thrust technique (see Chapter 2, page 38) and make sure the person is breathing. If you are unable to keep the airway open using the jaw thrust, turn the person carefully into the recovery position (see Chapter 2, page 31). If the person is not breathing start resuscitation (see Chapter 2, page 33).

key skills

If you suspect a person has a spinal injury, stop the event. Keep the person still, reassure him and call for an ambulance.

summary

Without the use of an X-ray or scan, it is impossible to accurately diagnose whether an injury is a sprain, strain, a fracture or a dislocation.

If you are in doubt, treat the injury as a fracture. Avoid moving the person and, if possible, reassure and support the injury while you are waiting for an ambulance. Do not give the person anything to eat or drink.

self-testers

1 A sprain tends to occur in:

a a muscle
b a joint
c a bone
d all of the above

2 What is the RICE procedure?

3 When taking a person with a fractured collarbone to hospital, you should:

a lay him on his side
b lay him on his back
c lay him in the recovery position
d sit him up

4 In the event of an open fracture, you should keep the wound:

a exposed to the air to clot

b covered to stop bleeding and keep the bone clean

c clean by rinsing with water

d elevated to stop bleeding

answers

1 **b**

2 **R**est, **I**ce, **C**ompress and **E**levate

3 **d**

4 **b**

6

winter sports

The popularity of winter sports such as skiing, ice-skating, sledging and snowboarding means that we have dedicated this chapter to the kinds of injuries and conditions that occur most commonly when undertaking such activities. We recognize that some of the injuries associated with this type of sport like sprains, strains and fractures are covered elsewhere in this book and we have not repeated the first-aid advice here.

Before we talk about the specific injuries and conditions associated with winter sports, there are a few considerations that will help to prevent some of the injuries described later in the chapter. Choice of clothing is very important when undertaking winter sports. There are many specialist-clothing manufacturers who design clothing for this purpose. If using non-specialist clothing, you should wear several thin layers rather than one thick layer. It is also important to keep your head covered as the body loses significant amount of heat through the head.

Ensure you have eaten prior to undertaking your sport and carry a snack and some fluids with you. Remember sunglasses and sunscreen when participating in winter sports. If you do undertake the activity alone, make sure someone knows where you are going and how long for.

hypothermia

This is a condition that occurs when there is prolonged exposure to cold resulting in a drop in the body's temperature. Hypothermia in its severest form can be fatal and it is important to remember that it can result from exposure to cold air or immersion in cold water.

If a person is suffering from hypothermia he will be cold to touch and the skin will be dry and pale. The person may be shivering but this may not be continuous. This shivering can appear to be quite dramatic and almost violent. The person may also appear dazed and confused and begin to lose consciousness. His breathing will be slow and shallow.

Your aim when treating hypothermia is to stop the person losing any more body heat, and to re-warm the person slowly. The most effective way to stop heat loss is to remove any wet clothing and replace it with dry clothing. Ensure the person is not lying directly on the cold ground. Lay him on some thick vegetation or some clothing. Cover with sleeping bags or blankets. A foil blanket is ideal as it helps prevent heat loss by radiating the heat back to the body. Ensure the person's head is covered throughout the treatment. You should give him some warm fluids to drink and some high-energy foods like chocolate to eat. Do not allow the person to drink alcohol. Alcohol opens up the blood vessels in the body by making them wider. This includes the blood vessels in the skin, so heat escapes and this could make the condition worse.

We do not recommend you put the person too close to a heater or fire or place a hot water bottle directly onto the skin because the body's blood will be diverted to the skin and away from the vital organs such as the brain. There are various types of heat pack available that can be used to heat the hands, feet or can be placed under the armpits.

key skills

When treating hypothermia, you should warm the person slowly, give warm drinks and high-energy foods and seek medical advice if necessary.

one-minute wonder

Q Why do you say not to give the person alcohol?

A Alcohol dilates the blood vessels and this can make the condition worse and make re-warming the person more difficult.

A person with severe hypothermia may be unconscious and not responding to you. It may be difficult to detect a pulse or check if the person is breathing. He will appear cold to touch and the skin may appear blue. These are the signs many people associate with death. Some people totally immersed in very cold water, especially those who are young, have been known to recover after as long as one hour in the water. As a result of this, you must start resuscitation unless the person is known to have been dead for some time.

In all cases, you should seek medical advice or call for an ambulance.

key skills

If a person is suffering from hypothermia, remove wet clothing and replace with dry. Warm him up, give chocolate and warm drinks and seek medical advice or call for an ambulance.

frostbite

This condition often occurs as a result of exposure to cold. It tends to affect the tips of the fingers and toes. Frostbite can occur even when these areas are covered by gloves or footwear. This condition is less common on the cheeks and ear lobes.

With frostbite, the affected area can be cold and complain of numbness and the skin appears hard and stiff. As the condition progresses the skin can look blotchy and blue.

Your aim as a first aider is to warm up the area by firstly removing gloves or boots or any jewellery that may be obstructing blood circulation. Then warm the part with your hands or by placing the digits in the person's armpits. If the frostbite affects the toes, you can place them in your friends or the first aider's armpits. You can also place the affected area in a bowl of warm water. You should dry the area and apply a gauze dressing. You should not put the frostbitten area close to direct heat or allow the person to drink alcohol.

Once the initial treatment has been provided, seek medical advice or take the person to hospital. In some cases the person with frostbite may also have hypothermia.

key skills

To treat frostbitten fingers, you should warm them slowly by placing them in the person's armpit. For toes, you can immerse in warm but not hot water. Do not give alcohol to drink or place to close to direct heat.

trenchfoot

This is a condition that results from exposure to wet and cool conditions. It usually results from wet feet in winter conditions but there have been reports of trenchfoot occurring in warmer conditions. Those involved in boating and canoeing activities are at risk.

To treat trenchfoot, you should remove the footwear and dry the feet. You should then slowly warm the feet, but do not put them directly in front of heat. Try and avoid walking if possible and put on clean dry socks and change them at least once a day.

key skills

To treat trenchfoot, you should remove footwear, dry the feet, slowly warm them and put on dry, warm, clean socks.

summary

Cold weather presents some obvious risks to sporting enthusiasts. However, many of the injuries and conditions that occur can be avoided by taking simple precautions. In the event of having to treat another person, always ensure your own safety and don't end up as a victim of the climate.

self-testers

1 In the case of hypothermia the person's skin will be:

a warm, wet and flushed

b cold, dry and pale

c red and damp

d flushed and dry

2 When treating frostbite, which of the following should you not do?

a place the affected area in hot water

b place the affected area in warm water

c place the affected area in direct heat

d give the person alcohol

answers

1 **b**

2 **a, c** and **d**

7

medical problems

In this chapter we will look at medical problems that people suffer from in an ongoing way, which can potentially affect their sporting performance. We will also examine those that happen suddenly while a person is playing sport. Some problems such as asthma and epilepsy, that have sudden events as part of their pattern, will overlap between the two groups. Others such as heart attacks fall exclusively into the second group.

asthma

Asthma is a medical problem that causes difficulty with breathing. During an asthma attack the muscles of the air passages in the lungs tighten and the linings of the air passages swell. This has the effect of narrowing the passages and therefore making it difficult to breathe.

Sometimes there is a recognized trigger for an attack but at other times there is no apparent reason. Triggers include cigarette smoke, having a cold and allergy to a substance such as pollen or a drug.

one-minute wonder

Q Can a person who suffers with asthma play outdoor sport?

A Yes, but it is important to recognize a trigger if playing field sports in summer, for example, as the personal trigger factor might be pollen, which may set off an asthmatic attack.

There is some debate over whether or not exercise triggers asthma, but it seems likely that some climatic conditions are relevant. Running in the open air is a greater stimulus to airway narrowing than running on an indoor treadmill and cold, dry air causes more narrowing than warm, moist air.

recognizing asthma

A person suffering from an asthma attack will have difficulty with breathing, especially breathing out. There will be a cough, wheezing and some distress depending upon the severity of the attack. With a severe attack there will also be difficulty speaking and blueness around the lips and fingernails, which indicates a lack of oxygen in the body.

Normally, a person who suffers from attacks of asthma will be aware of the problem and have a reliever inhaler. This should be taken as soon as an attack starts. If a person is actively taking part in a sporting activity he should stop what he is doing and rest, keep calm and take his inhaler. He should also try to breathe slowly and deeply. The inhaler should relieve the attack after a few minutes. If it does not, he should take the inhaler again.

how to use an inhaler

The inhaler is taken by mouth. The inhaler must be shaken to mix the drug inside with the propellant and when the cap is removed make sure the mouthpiece is clean. When the person is ready he should place his mouth around the inhaler and co-ordinate activating the inhaler with taking a slow deep breath. He should try to breathe in and hold his breath to a count of ten and then breathe out. If available, he may wish to use a spacer device. To use this, the drug is puffed into the spacer and the person breathes normally in and out from the spacer. He should breathe in as soon as possible after the drug is puffed into the spacer.

key skills

If the person has an asthma attack when playing sport, he should stop and use his inhaler. If the attack does not respond to treatment, call for an ambulance.

one-minute wonder

Q Can I take someone else's inhaler if I have left mine at home?

A This is not good practice as it is unhygienic and it may not be the same inhaler. However, if you recognize it as the same inhaler you usually use and you are willing to take the hygiene risk then you can use another person's inhaler if outside help is not readily available.

Unfortunately, not all asthma attacks respond to treatment and it is important to recognize when a person is not improving after taking the reliever inhaler and then to call for an ambulance. This will be necessary when the inhaler has had no effect after five minutes, when the person's breathing is getting worse, when breathlessness makes talking difficult and when the person is exhausted.

epilepsy

This is a medical condition in which a person suffers from seizures. A seizure is the result of an electrical disturbance in the brain and is a sudden and dramatic event that can take everyone by surprise. Very often, people who have epilepsy carry a warning card or wear a medical-alert bracelet or necklace. A person who suffers repeated seizures often has a sense when a seizure is coming on, so when playing sport, this gives the person a short time to move out of the sporting arena and away from any danger.

recognizing a seizure

A seizure follows a pattern. There will be a sudden loss of consciousness and the person may let out a cry. This will be followed by body stiffness, then jerking movements that can be quite violent, possibly accompanied by urinary incontinence and biting of the tongue. At the end of the seizure the muscles will relax and the person returns to normal but because a seizure is an unnerving experience the person may well feel tired, disorientated and wish to sleep.

helping a person who is having a seizure

If possible, ease the person's fall but do not put yourself at risk. Keep calm and try to stop other team colleagues or bystanders from rushing to the person to try to help. Let the seizure take its course and make sure the person doesn't hurt himself. If possible, place some soft padding under the head, loosen tight clothing and protect the person as much as you can. When the seizure has stopped make sure the person is breathing and place him in the recovery position (see Chapter 2).

Remain with the person until he is fully recovered and has someone to take him home and be there with him. If this is not possible, make sure the person goes to a place of safety where he is accompanied. Do not let him drive.

Call an ambulance if the seizure lasts for more than five minutes, this is the person's first seizure, the person remains unconscious for more than ten minutes after the seizure, the person sustains other injuries or consciousness is not regained between seizures.

key skills

If you encounter a person having a seizure, move furniture or equipment so that he does not hurt himself. Loosen any tight clothing. Once the active phase of the seizure is over, place him in the recovery position to rest.

one-minute wonder

Q Are there things I shouldn't do when a person is having a seizure?

A You must not try to stop the seizure by restraining the person because it will not be possible and may cause other injuries. You must not put anything into the person's mouth or give him anything to eat or drink because he may choke.

diabetes

Diabetes is a medical problem that arises when the body is unable to regulate the blood sugar because there is a lack of the hormone that usually regulates the sugar, known as insulin. There are two types of diabetes: Type 1 and Type 2. Type 1 usually appears early in life and is the result of a failure of the insulin-producing cells in the body. It requires the use of insulin injections for the rest of the person's life. Type 2 diabetes usually comes on later in life and is the result of the body not producing enough insulin. It can usually be controlled by diet and medication. The aim is to balance the amount of sugar in the body with the amount of insulin, in order to keep a steady level of circulating blood sugar.

When the insulin–sugar balance is disturbed and there is very little sugar in the blood this is known as hypoglycaemia and when there is too much sugar this is known as hyperglycaemia.

Diabetes-related problems in sport are usually to do with hypoglycaemia. For example, the school pupil, who is late getting up one morning, doesn't have breakfast but remembers to take his insulin and then plays sport before eating again. Because he didn't have breakfast he hasn't put any sugar into his body for the insulin to work on and then by playing sport he further reduces his blood sugar to dangerous levels and hypoglycaemia is likely.

recognizing a hypoglycaemic attack

As the person's blood sugar falls he might feel an attack coming on. He will feel dizzy, faint, hungry and sweaty. He may act irrationally and feel confused, his pulse and breathing will be fast and if the low blood sugar is not reversed he will lose consciousness.

action to take

The aim of treatment is to raise the blood sugar by giving the person a sugary drink or a high carbohydrate food. If the person carries glucose tablets or a sugary gel these can be used. Giving sugar as soon as possible should reverse the hypoglycaemia and revive the person until he is able to have more food to restore his diabetic balance.

Do not, however, give food or drink if the person has lost, or is rapidly losing, consciousness as this can lead to him choking.

key skills

In the event of a person becoming hypoglycaemic, you should try and raise the blood sugar by giving a sugary drink or glucose tablets. If the person falls unconscious, call for an ambulance.

one-minute wonder

Q How can I tell the difference between hypoglycaemia and hyperglycaemia?

A This can be difficult, but remember in sport the most likely problem is going to be hypoglycaemia and so always give sugar to an ill diabetic person. You will quickly correct hypoglycaemia and cause little harm if he is suffering from hyperglycaemia.

5 5

heart attacks

A heart attack occurs without warning and is caused by a blood clot that causes a blockage in an artery carrying blood to part of the heart muscle. This blockage is known as a coronary thrombosis and its effect depends on how much of the heart muscle is damaged. The main danger with a heart attack is that the heart will go into an abnormal rhythm and stop beating. If the heart stops this is known as a cardiac arrest.

recognizing a heart attack

If you ask the person how he is feeling, he will usually tell you he has a crushing pain in the central part of his chest with the pain sometimes going into the arms, the jaw or the back.

He will also have a sense that he is very ill and be breathless, faint and nauseated. He will look ashen and have cold, clammy skin.

how to help

As soon as you suspect a heart attack call for an ambulance so that the person receives medical help as soon as possible. Tell the operator you suspect a heart attack. You should also encourage the person to rest the heart by sitting as quietly as possible in a comfortable position. Ideally this will be sitting down, leaning against a wall or chair with his head and shoulders supported and his knees bent. If the person has medication such as aspirin or an aerosol for angina help him to take it and do not leave the person unless you need to call an ambulance, as he may have a cardiac arrest and collapse at any time. If he does collapse you will need to perform resuscitation (see Chapter 2).

key skills

If you suspect a person is having a heart attack, ask him to take an aspirin or other medication he may have. Sit him down and call for an ambulance. Be prepared to resuscitate.

sudden death

Fortunately sudden death in sport is rare but it can happen. Most sudden deaths in sport are caused by heart problems and by far the most common condition leading to sudden death during exercise in the over-35 age group is coronary artery disease. In the younger age group it is very rare and usually a result of an abnormality of the heart that has been present since birth and which reaches a critical point when the heart can no longer work normally.

People are at greatest risk when taking part in extreme exertion sports such as marathon running, cross-country running, skiing, basketball, football, hockey and track sports.

recognizing a sudden death situation

The person will suddenly collapse to the ground. There will have been no warning signs. He will be unconscious, have no breathing and no signs of circulation.

action to take

Call for an ambulance immediately. Start resuscitation.

summary

Many people with medical conditions lead full and active lives and undertake strenuous sporting activities without any problems. However, there are conditions like diabetes and asthma where undertaking exercise needs to be carefully planned to avoid or reduce risks. If you are considering participating in any new sporting activity and are already taking medication, you should check with your doctor before commencing.

It is possible to confuse the pain associated with a heart attack with a severe attack of indigestion or a muscle strain in the chest. If in doubt, you should always seek advice.

self-testers

1 Trigger factors for asthma include:

a pollen
b cold, dry air
c cigarette smoke
d certain drugs
e having a cold

2 **When looking after a person you suspect is having a heart attack you should:**

a wait to see if the pain gets worse before calling the ambulance

b make sure the person rests

c allow the person to continue the activity

d make the person lie down

e give the person any medication he may have

3 **When looking after a person who is having a seizure you should:**

a try to open the airway

b move the person out of the sporting arena

c try to stop the seizure by restraining the person

d remove any dangerous hazards from around the person

e stay with the person after the seizure is over

4 **Signs of hypoglycaemia include:**

a warm, moist skin

b hunger

c confused behaviour

d slow pulse rate

e rapid breathing

5 **What do the letters AVPU stand for?**

answers

1 **a, b, c, d** and **e**

2 **b** and **e**

3 **d** and **e**

4 **a, b, c** and **e**

5 **A**lert; responds to **V**oice; responds to **P**ain; **U**nresponsive

case studies

Ernie's story

Ernest Jones was an enthusiastic rather than capable golfer. Easter Monday 2001 had started like any other Monday. Ernie left home at 6.45 a.m. as he routinely did to join two other recently retired colleagues for nine holes followed by a spot of breakfast.

'I usually had a piece of toast when leaving the house and a glass of orange juice', said Ernie. However, on this morning Ernie did not feel hungry. On arrival at the club he began to feel a bit dizzy and thought it was just down to the fact that he had not eaten. The smell of cooked bacon coming from the restaurant was difficult to resist so he suggested to his playing partners that on this occasion they break with tradition and have a bacon roll and coffee before starting the round.

'At the first tee, I thought the roll and coffee had done the trick and I was feeling a little better', said Ernie. However, on arrival at the seventh hole the dizziness had returned, but now it was accompanied by shortness of breath and a feeling of sickness. By the time he arrived at the eighth hole, Ernie was feeling so unwell he had to sit down. One playing partner suggested that one of them should return to the clubhouse to get a motorized buggy to take Ernie back. It was now clear to Ernie and his playing colleague that his condition was getting worse and he was now beginning to feel 'a weight on his chest'. One of his friends immediately recognized that all the signs and symptoms added up to the fact that he'd had a heart attack.

Luckily, George, Ernie's long-term playing partner, had broken the club rules and had his mobile phone with him although it was not switched on. 'I dialled 999 for an ambulance', said George, 'but I must admit, I felt a bit stupid giving the address of the incident as the eighth-hole on the western course at Lira Golf club.'

While they waited for the ambulance to arrive, John, Ernie's other playing partner, and the green keeper had returned in the buggy. 'We were not sure whether we should move him and drive back to the clubhouse and wait for the ambulance, or leave him where he was until the ambulance arrived', said George. The green keeper returned to the clubhouse to show the ambulance crew where the ambulance was required and how to access it via a service road. 'By the time the ambulance arrived, I had never seen a man so pale. He had the look of death, slumped over his golf trolley but still trying to be brave despite the pain he was feeling in his chest', said George.

The ambulance crew immediately gave Ernie oxygen, set up a drip and gave him some drugs. Ernie spent just under two weeks in hospital but five months away from the golf course. 'Thankfully, my game didn't get any worse in those five months', says Ernie.

authors' observations

This story highlights the importance of making an early call to the ambulance service, especially if the location of the incident is not easily accessible. In this case Ernie was fortunate that one of his friends had his mobile phone with him and his playing partner identified that he was sufficiently unwell to require an ambulance. The dilemma the bystanders faced was whether to move him to a point on the course where he would receive expert care more quickly or to leave him where he was. It is very difficult to be definitive about what to do but in this case, leaving him where he was turned out to be the right decision.

This case also highlights the fact that the onset of a heart attack is not always obvious and can be confused with a general feeling of being unwell. In this case, the condition gradually got worse and it was not until Ernie started complaining of pains in his chest, combined with the other signs and symptoms, that George suspected a heart attack.

Kate's story

Kate Douglas has been an Arsenal supporter all her life (24 years). Being the only girl in the family meant that playing with her brothers inevitably meant football. She became very good. At the age of 13, she represented her county but moving away to study Sports Psychology at university meant that playing sport had to compete with her studies. She still enjoyed the competitiveness of playing but had resigned herself to the fact that the chance of playing professional sport had passed her by.

It was while playing in a mixed five-a-side tournament with a group of students from the university that she received what she describes as 'my biggest break in sport'. 'I cannot even blame the boys in the opposing team for being over competitive, as it was a challenge with one of the female opponents that caused the injury. It was a 50:50 ball and I overstretched to reach the ball and the girl on the opposing team did likewise. Unfortunately, when attempting to clear the ball, she caught my ankle.' Kate knew it was a bad tackle but did not realize the damage it had done. Kate had received many football injuries over the years and initially did not suspect this was more serious than some bruising.

'I tried to stand up', said Kate 'and it was then that I realized something was definitely wrong. The pain was excruciating. It must have sounded like I had been shot.' Kate immediately sat down on the astro turf and the game stopped. One of the teammates began to examine her ankle. 'I couldn't stand him even touching my leg due to the discomfort, but thinking back on it, I was probably still in denial, thinking it was a bad sprain.'

Once the sock had been removed it was obvious there was some kind of injury as the area around the ankle appeared swollen and red. Two of Kate's friends carried her from the pitch. 'As they were doing so, I thought my foot was moving too much and, even though I was not putting any weight on it, the pain was still very bad.'

Kate's friends loaded her into the car and the pain was now unbearable. On arrival at the hospital, Kate was immediately placed on a trolley with her leg elevated and ice packs around her ankle. X-rays confirmed a fractured ankle. Initially, hospital staff thought she might require an operation to mend the damage. The ankle was immobilized for three months and it gradually improved. Now three years later, Kate still has stiffness and discomfort in the ankle. She has not played competitive football since that day.

authors' observations

By reading this story we can almost feel the pain and discomfort Kate was in. As we have said earlier, without an X-ray, it is often difficult to tell the difference between a sprain and a strain, or a fracture.

In this case, Kate was clearly in a lot of pain. There was evidence of some swelling but the bystanders were not sure how significant the swelling was.

A good way to measure the amount of swelling is to compare the injured ankle to the uninjured one. On this occasion, it may have indicated the seriousness of the injury. You should never ignore a person's complaints of pain. In this case, applying ice to the injury as quickly as possible would have reduced the amount of pain and swelling. The fact that even when being carried, Kate was still experiencing pain, suggests that on this occasion it may have been better to leave her on the pitch and call the ambulance service.

Andrew's story

Andrew was looking forward to Saturday afternoon's match. He had been training hard and had finally made it into his local town's 1st XV rugby team. The team was doing well and during the season had steadily improved its position in the local league.

Andrew's position in the team was hooker and he felt he was well supported by his team mates in the rest of the pack, most of whom were much more experienced players than him.

All was going well in the game, Andrew was playing well, and his team was leading by 10 points to 3 after about 30 minutes of the game. An infringement occurred and his team was awarded the put in at a scrum. The two teams engaged but suddenly the scrum collapsed and Andrew fell awkwardly onto his head with a member of the second row on top of him. At this point he thinks he "blacked out" for a few seconds because when he came round, he was lying on the pitch where the scrum had collapsed and he had tingling sensations in his arms and legs. He wanted to get up to make sure his arms and legs were still working properly but one of his teammates was holding his head and another one was holding his hand and telling him very firmly that he must lay still. He knew the one who was holding his head had very large hands and he felt his head was in a vice-like grip. He couldn't move.

After what felt like an age the ambulance arrived, strapped him onto a rigid, cold board with his head between two blocks and took him to hospital. Andrew was fortunate – despite the early tingling feelings, there was no serious damage to his neck and he made a full recovery.

authors' observations

Andrew was lucky. It is possible to protect the head from injury by wearing a helmet or skullcap but it is so difficult to protect the neck in impact sports such as rugby. Other sports such as horse riding, cycling and motor sport present a definite risk when being thrown off, especially if travelling at speed.

Andrew's teammates knew exactly what to do and did it well. They didn't move Andrew, they didn't let him try to get up, in fact they told him to lie still and one of them held his head in a firm grip so that his neck didn't move. It is sometimes difficult to persuade others that the game must be stopped and the injured person not moved to the side of the pitch but this is vitally important and seems to have been done in this case. It is also difficult to know whether or not Andrew would have suffered lasting damage if he had been moved but it is not worth taking that risk. Everything was done to prevent this, and thankfully in Andrew's case it worked.

first-aid kit contents

There are no hard and fast rules about what should be in your personal first-aid kit. What you are most likely to need will depend on where you are and what you are doing. For example, on the sports field or in the gym, ice packs would be more commonly used than in other scenarios. We recommend that you keep a fully-stocked kit at home and in your car.

Here are some core items that we recommend you have in any kit:

- **plasters in assorted sizes** – these are applied to small cuts and grazes. Covering the wound with a clean, dry dressing will help prevent the area from becoming infected as well as help to stop any bleeding.
- **sterile wound dressings in assorted sizes** – these are used for wounds such as cuts or burns. Place the dressing pad over the injured area, making sure that the pad is larger than the wound. Then wrap the roller bandage around the limb to secure it.
- **triangular bandages** – commonly used for slings, these are strong supportive bandages. If they are sterile then they can also be used as dressings for wounds and burns.
- **safety pins** – useful for securing crêpe bandages and triangular bandages.

- **adhesive tape** – useful to hold and secure bandages comfortably in place. Some people are allergic to the adhesive, but hypoallergenic tape is available.
- **sterile gauze swabs** – these can be used to clean around a wound or in conjunction with other bandages and tape to help keep wounds clean and dry.
- **non-alcoholic cleansing wipes** – useful for cleaning cuts and grazes. They can also be used to clean your hands if water and soap are not available.
- **roller bandages** – used to give support to injured joints, to secure dressings in place, to maintain pressure on them, and to limit swelling.
- **disposable gloves** – these single-use gloves are an important safety measure to avoid infecting wounds as well as to protect you.
- **scissors** – using a round-ended pair of scissors will not cause injury and will make short work of cutting dressings or bandages to size. It is useful to have a strong pair that will cut through clothing.
- **insect repellent** – a protective spray against insect bites. Always follow the instructions provided. Never use repellents over cuts, wounds or irritated skin.
- **foil survival blanket** – this blanket provides protection from hypothermia caused by exposure to the elements and conserves body heat in cases of shock and trauma.
- **rehydration sachet** – to replace lost fluids and salts, dissolve a sachet in water and drink. This gives fast and effective replacement of body fluids during illness.

- **burn gel** – use directly on a burn to cool and relieve the pain of minor burns and to help prevent infection. Very useful if water is not available.
- **ice pack** – cooling an injury and the surrounding area can reduce swelling and pain. Always wrap an ice pack in a dry cloth and do not use it for more than ten minutes at one application.
- **tweezers** – useful for picking out splinters.
- **thermometer** – used to assess the body temperature. There are several different types including the traditional glass mercury thermometer and digital thermometer, as well as the forehead thermometer and the ear sensor. Normal body temperature is 37°C (98.6°F).
- **face shield or pocket mask** (a hygiene shield for giving rescue breaths) – these are plastic barriers with a reinforced hole to fit over the person's mouth. Use the shield to protect you and the person from infections when giving rescue breaths.
- **note pad and pen** – use the pad to record any information about the injured person that may be of use to the emergency services when they arrive. For example, the name and address of the person, how the accident occurred, and any observations. It is also useful to record vital signs so that you can monitor how well the person is doing over a period of time.
- **basic first-aid information** – a basic guide to first-aid tips, and emergency information (you can use the first aid essentials pull-out card in this book).

This is not an exhaustive list and there are many more items you may find useful to add to your kit. What is vital is that you have the necessary supplies ready to hand for when you need them.

Many people like to keep items such as antiseptic cream in their kits. The British Red Cross does not include anything which may no longer be sterile after the first use because of the risk of infection and allergies.

It is easy to make your own first-aid kit by collecting the items listed above or, alternatively, you could simply buy a complete kit. For more information on British Red Cross kits visit **www.redcross.org.uk/firstaidproducts** or call 0845 601 7105.

The Health and Safety Executive (HSE) is responsible for the regulation of almost all the risks to health and safety arising from work activity in Britain. Regulations concerning kit contents do apply to employers. For more information about first-aid kits and training for the workplace visit **www.redcrossfirstaidtraining.co.uk** or call 0870 170 9110.

household first-aid equipment

Throughout this book we have made reference to the importance of having first-aid skills, knowledge and equipment. In terms of equipment, we recommend you have a well-stocked first-aid kit (see page 117), but we also recognize that there are emergency situations where you will not have access to any of the equipment. In such situations you will have to be creative and use whatever equipment is available to you. In this section we have identified some of the items most of us already have in our homes and suggest how they can be useful in a first-aid situation.

- **beer** – you may not always have access to cold running water when treating a burn or scald. In this case, use some other cold liquid like beer, soft drink or milk. The aim is to cool the burnt area as quickly as possible using whatever cold liquid is available. Beer can be used to cool the area while waiting for water or while walking the person to a supply of cold running water. Remember, the area should be cooled for at least ten minutes for the treatment to be effective.
- **chair** – a chair has numerous first-aid uses; when treating a nosebleed, sit the person down while pinching the nose and tilting the head forward. If you are treating a bleed from a large wound to the leg, you should lay the person down and raise the leg above the level of the heart. A chair is ideal for this purpose.

- **chocolate** – chocolate can be given to a conscious person who is diabetic and having a hypoglycaemia attack known as a “hypo”. This can help raise the person’s blood sugar. Chocolate can also be given to a person with hypothermia as high-energy foods will help to warm the person up.
- **cling film** – cling film can be used to wrap around a burn or a scald once it has cooled. It is an ideal covering as it does not stick to the burn. It also keeps the burnt area clean and because it is transparent, you can continue to monitor the burn without removing the covering.
- **credit card** – when an insect sting is visible on the skin, a credit card can be used to scrape it away. Using the edge of the credit card, drag it across the skin. This will remove the sting. Using a credit card is preferable to using a pair of tweezers as some stings contain a sac of poison and if the sting is grasped with tweezers you may inject the sac of poison into the skin. If you do not have a credit card you can use the back of a kitchen knife or any other object similar to a credit card.
- **food bag** – a clean freezer or sandwich bag makes an ideal cover for a burn or scald to the hand. The injured part should be placed in the bag once the cooling has finished. By placing it in the bag you reduce the risk of infection and it also helps reduce the level of pain.
- **frozen peas** – frozen peas or other frozen small fruit and vegetables can be used to treat a sprain or strain. Wrap the peas in a tea towel or something similar and place them onto the injury. This will help to reduce pain and swelling. Peas are

ideal as they can be moulded around the injury more easily than bigger fruit and vegetables.

- **milk** – if an adult tooth is dislodged and cannot be placed back in its socket, it should be placed in a container of milk. This will stop it drying out and increase the possibility of it being successfully replanted by a dental surgeon.
- **paper bag** – a panic attack often results in the person hyperventilating (breathing very quickly). Reassure the person and get them to breath into a paper bag, this will help to regulate and slow down the persons breathing.
- **steam** – if a child has an attack of croup, run the tap in the bathroom to create a steamy atmosphere, this can help to relieve the symptoms.
- **vinegar** – if a person is stung by a tropical jellyfish, pour vinegar over the site of the sting. This will help to stop the poison spreading around the body.
- **water** – cold running water is the preferred treatment for burns and scalds. Place the burn under a cold water tap as quickly as possible and leave it there for at least ten minutes.
- **Yellow Pages and a broom** – in the event of having to provide assistance to a person with an electrical injury, where the person is attached to the current, you can stand on a copy of the Yellow Pages to insulate yourself from an electrical shock. You should then move the electrical cable away using a dry piece of wood, a broom handle is ideal.

about the Red Cross

the British Red Cross and the International Red Cross and Red Crescent Movement

The British Red Cross is a leading UK charity with 40,000 volunteers working in almost every community. We provide a range of high-quality services in local communities across the UK every day. We respond to emergencies, train first aiders, help vulnerable people regain their independence, and assist refugees and asylum seekers.

The British Red Cross is part of the International Red Cross and Red Crescent Movement, the world's largest independent humanitarian organization. This Movement comprises three components: the International Committee of the Red Cross; the International Federation of Red Cross and Red Crescent Societies; and 181 National Red Cross and National Red Crescent Societies around the world.

As a member of the International Red Cross and Red Crescent Movement, the British Red Cross is committed to, and bound by, its Fundamental Principles:

- Humanity
- Impartiality
- Neutrality
- Independence
- Voluntary service
- Unity
- Universality.

the International Committee of the Red Cross

Based in Geneva, Switzerland, the International Committee of the Red Cross (ICRC) is a private, independent humanitarian institution, whose role is defined as part of the Geneva Conventions. Serving as a neutral intermediary during international wars and civil conflicts, it provides protection and assistance for civilians, prisoners of war and the wounded, and provides a similar function during internal disturbances.

To find out more visit **www.icrc.org**

the International Federation of Red Cross and Red Crescent Societies

Also based in Geneva, the Federation is a separately constituted body that co-ordinates international relief provided by National Societies for victims of natural disasters, and for refugees and displaced persons outside conflict zones. It also assists Red Cross and Red Crescent Societies with their own development, helping them to plan and implement disaster preparedness and development projects on behalf of vulnerable people in local communities.

To find out more visit **www.ifrc.org**

National Red Cross and National Red Crescent Societies

In most countries around the world, there exists a National Red Cross or Red Crescent Society. Each Society has a responsibility to help vulnerable people within its own borders, and to work in conjunction with the Movement to protect and support those in crisis worldwide.

To find out more about the British Red Cross visit **www.redcross.org.uk**

taking it further

useful addresses

NHS Direct
www.nhsdirect.nhs.uk
Tel: 0845 4647

NHS Direct Sport Injuries
www.nhsdirect.nhs.uk/en.asp?TopicID=619&AreaID=4083&LinkID=3158

Sport Development Website
www.sportdevelopment.org.uk
A collection of resources about sport development in the UK.

Sport England
www.sportengland.org
3rd floor, Victoria House, Bloomsbury Square,
London, WC1B 4SE
Tel: 0845 850 8508
Provide strategic lead for sport in England and develop the Government's objectives. Encourages people to get involved in sport.

Sport England Lottery Fund
Tel: 0845 7649649

The International Federation of Sports Medicine
www.fims.org/fims/frames.asp
An international organization comprised of individual members, national associations, and multinational groups, with a common involvement with sports medicine on all continents.

International Red Cross contact details

Australia
National Office, 155 Pelham Street, 3053 Carlton VIC
Tel: switchboard (61) (3) 93451800
Fax: (61) (3) 93482513
E-mail: redcross@nat.redcross.org.au
www.redcross.org.au

Canada
170 Metcalfe Street, Suite 300 Ottawa, Ontario K2P 2P2
Tel: (1) (613) 7401900
Fax: (1) (613) 7401911
Telex: CANCROSS 05-33784
E-mail: cancross@redcross.ca
www.redcross.ca

Hong Kong
3 Harcourt Road, Wanchai, Hong Kong
Tel: (852) 28020021
E-mail: hcs@redcross.org.hk
www.redcross.org.hk

India
Red Cross, Building 1, Red Cross Road, 110001 New Delhi
Tel: (91) (112) 371 64 24
Fax: (91) (112) 371 74 54
E-mail: indcross@vsnl.com
www.indianredcross.org

Malaysia
JKR 32, Jalan Nipah, Off Jalan Ampang, 55000 Kuala Lumpur
Tel: (60) (3) 42578122/42578236/42578348/
42578159/42578227
Fax: (60) (3) 42533191
E-mail: mrcs@po.jaring.my
www.redcrescent.org.my

New Zealand
69 Molesworth Street, Thorndon, Wellington
Tel: (64) (4) 4723750
Fax: (64) (4) 4730315
E-mail: national@redcross.org.nz
www.redcross.org.nz

Singapore
Red Cross House, 15 Penang Lane, 238486 Singapore
Tel: (65) 6 3360269
Fax: (65) 6 3374360
E-mail: redcross@starhub.net.sg
www.redcross.org.sg

South Africa
1st Floor, Helen Bowden Building, Beach Road, Granger Bay,
8002 Cape Town
Tel: (27) (21) 4186640
Fax: (27) (21) 4186644
E-mail: sarcs@redcross.org.za
www.redcross.org.za

Taiwan and China
No: 8 Beixingiao Santiao, Dongcheng, East City District, 100007
Beijing
Tel: (86) (10) 84025890
Fax: (86) (10) 6406 0566/9928
E-mail: rcsc@chineseredcross.org.cn
www.redcross.org.cn

index

5 minute first aid life-saving skills

- **Would you know what to do to save someone's life?**
- **Did you know that it is highly likely it will be someone close to you who will need your help?**
- **Do you want to be able to make a difference in an emergency?**

This could be the most important book you will ever read. *Five-Minute First Aid Life-Saving Skills* provides the reader with invaluable information and advice that will equip him/her with the skills needed to deal with an emergency, whether this be unconsciousness, cardiac arrest, major blood loss, choking or, most importantly, how to save a life.

What's stopping you? **£5.99**

British Red Cross
Caring for people in crisis

5 minute first aid for travel

- **Would you know what to do to save someone's life?**
- **Did you know that it is highly likely it will be someone close to you who will need your help?**
- **Do you want to be able to make a difference in an emergency?**

This could be the most important book you will ever read. *Five-Minute First Aid for Travel* will provide any traveller or individual working within the travel industry with invaluable information and advice, from the treatment of bites and stings, burns and fevers to dehydration, hypothermia and, most importantly, how to save a life.

What's stopping you? **£6.99**

British Red Cross
Caring for people in crisis